High-Yield Neuroanatomy

High-Yield Neuroanatomy

James D. Fix, Ph.D.
Professor of Anatomy
Department of Anatomy
Marshall University
School of Medicine
Huntington, West Virginia

Williams & Wilkins
BALTIMORE • PHILADELPHIA • HONG KONG
LONDON • MUNICH • SYDNEY • TOKYO
A Waverly Company

Williams & Wilkins

Acquisitions Editor: Elizabeth A. Nieginski
Development Editor: Donna Rae Siegfried
Project Editor: Amy G. Dinkel
Production Coordinator: Peter J. Carley
Illustrator: Patricia MacAllen

Copyright © 1995
Williams & Wilkins
Suite 5025
Rose Tree Corporate Center–Bldg. II
1400 N. Providence Road
Media, PA 19063-2043 USA

Printed in the United States of America

Library of Congress Cataloging-in-Publication Data

Fix, James D.
    High-yield neuroanatomy / James D. Fix.
        p.   cm. — (Board review series)
    Includes index.
    ISBN 0-683-03248-8
    1. Neuroanatomy—Outlines, syllabi, etc.   2. Neuroanatomy—
Examinations, questions, etc.   I. Title.   II. Series.
    [DNLM: 1. Nervous System—anatomy & histology—examination questions.
    2. Nervous System—anatomy & histology—outlines.   WL 18 F566h 1995]
QM451.F588   1994
611'.8'076—dc20
DNLM/DLC
for Library of Congress   94-44404
                                                                       CIP

                                                                97 98
                                                          5 6 7 8 9 10

Contents

Preface

High-Yield Neuroanatomy is neuroanatomy at its irreducible minimum and contains most, if not all, of the recurring national board themes. The sole purpose of the book is to get you through the nervous system topics covered on the USMLE Step 1. To make the most of this book, study the illustrations carefully and read the legends. Many board-type questions come from this source. In fact, the answers to at least 20 common USMLE questions are embedded within this preface. Remember these tips as you scan the chapters:

Chapter 1: The cross-sectional anatomy of this chapter provides you with the essential examination structures labeled on computed tomography scans and magnetic resonance images.

Chapter 2: CSF pathways are well-demonstrated in Figure 2-1. CSF is produced by the choroid plexus and absorbed by the arachnoid villi of the venous sinuses.

Chapter 3: The essential arteries and the functional areas irrigated by them are shown in this chapter. You may expect angiograms, such as those in Figures 3-4 and 3-5, to be on the examination.

Chapter 4: The neural crest and its derivatives, the dual origin of the pituitary gland, and the difference between spina bifida and the Arnold-Chiari malformation are presented in this chapter.

Chapter 5: Nerve cells contain Nissl substance in their perikarya and dendrites but not in their axons.

Chapter 6: The adult spinal cord terminates at the lower border of the first lumbar vertebra; the newborn's spinal cord extends to the third lumbar vertebra.

Chapter 7: Tracts of the spinal cord are reduced to four examination points: pyramidal tract, dorsal columns, pain and temperature, and Horner's tract.

Chapter 8: Two of the most important lesions of the spinal cord—Brown-Séquard syndrome and Lou Gehrig's disease—are presented in this chapter, as well as other lesions.

Chapter 9: The upper face division of the facial nucleus receives bilateral corticobulbar input. The lower face division of the facial nucleus receives contralateral corticobulbar input.

Chapter 10: In this chapter, you are reminded that CN V-1 is the afferent limb of the corneal reflex, and that CN V-1, CN V-2, CN III, CN IV, and CN VI are all found in the cavernous sinus. See Figure 10-2.

Chapter 11: Figure 11-1 shows the auditory pathway in a very simple but satisfactory sketch.

Chapter 12: This chapter teaches you the two types of vestibular nystagmus: postrotational nystagmus and caloric nystagmus (COWS). The MLF syndrome is a common USMLE item.

Chapter 13: This chapter on the cranial nerves is pivotal; it spawns more neuroanatomy examination questions than any other chapter. Carefully study Figures 13-2, 13-3, and 13-4; they are high-yield areas.

Chapter 14: The two most important syndromes caused by lesions of the brain stem—occlusion of the anterior spinal artery (Figure 14-1A) and occlusion of the posterior inferior cerebellar artery (Figure 14-1B)—are covered in this chapter.

Chapter 15: Figure 15-1 shows the most important cerebellar circuit. The inhibitory GABAergic Purkinje cells are paramount in this pathway.

Chapter 16: Figure 16-1 gives you all the information you need to know about what goes in and out of the thalamus—the "Grand Central Station" of the CNS.

Chapter 17: Figures 17-1 and 17-2 are key to understanding the visual system. Visual field defects are on every USMLE.

Chapter 18: The important anatomy of the autonomic nervous system is clearly seen in Figures 18-1 and 18-2.

Chapter 19: In Figure 19-1, you can see that the paraventricular and supraoptic nuclei synthesize and release ADH and oxytocin.

Chapter 20: Damage to the amygdala results in Klüver-Bucy syndrome. Damage to the hippocampus results in memory loss. Damage to the mamillary bodies results in Wernicke-Korsakoff syndrome. All of these are discussed in this chapter on the limbic system.

Chapter 21: Figure 21-3 shows you the important circuitry of the basal ganglia and their associated neurotransmitters. Parkinson's disease is associated with a loss of cells in the substantia nigra. Huntington's disease is associated with a loss of cells in the caudate nucleus. Hemiballism results from infarcts of the subthalamic nucleus.

Chapter 22: In this chapter, the pathways of the major neurotransmitters are illustrated simply in separate brain maps. Glutamate is the major excitatory transmitter of the brain; GABA is the major inhibitory transmitter of the brain.

Chapter 23: This chapter describes the important functional areas of the brain. Figure 23-4 shows the major hemispheric lesions of the dominant and nondominant hemispheres.

I wish you good luck.

James D. Fix

Acknowledgments

I wish to thank my medical students, colleagues, and members of the staff of Williams & Wilkins for their valuable comments, suggestions, and help. I especially would like to thank Donna Siegfried, Development Editor, for her perceptive editorial suggestions that have made this a more lucid presentation. I thank Patricia MacAllen for her fine illustrations, and Beth Goldner for her persistence, patience, and organization. Thanks also go to Jane Velker and Elizabeth Nieginski for their editorial direction.

1

Cross-Sectional Anatomy of the Brain

I. **INTRODUCTION.** The five illustrations in this chapter, which correspond with the following sections, represent a **mini-atlas** of brain slices in the three orthogonal planes (i.e., midsagittal, coronal, axial) used in computed tomography (CT) and magnetic resonance imaging (MRI) scans. An *insert* on the figures shows the level of the slice. The most commonly tested structures are listed for each cross-section.

II. **MIDSAGITTAL SECTION (Figure 1-1).** The location of the following structures should be known:

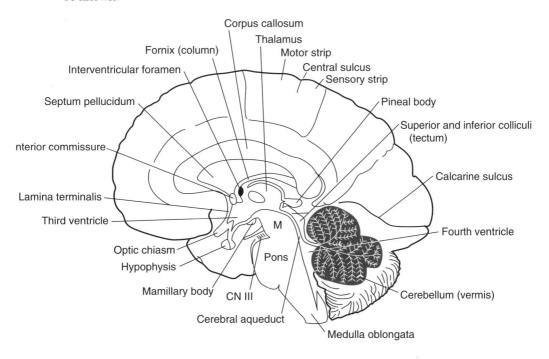

Figure 1-1. Midsagittal section of the brain and brain stem showing the structures surrounding the third and fourth ventricles. The brain stem includes the midbrain (*M*), the pons (*P*), and the medulla oblongata.

A. Anterior commissure

B. Cerebellar vermis

C. Cerebral aqueduct

D. Cranial nerve (CN) III

E. Corpus callosum

F. Fornix

G. Mamillary body

H. Optic chiasm

I. Pineal body

J. Pituitary gland (hypophysis)

K. Tectum (colliculi)

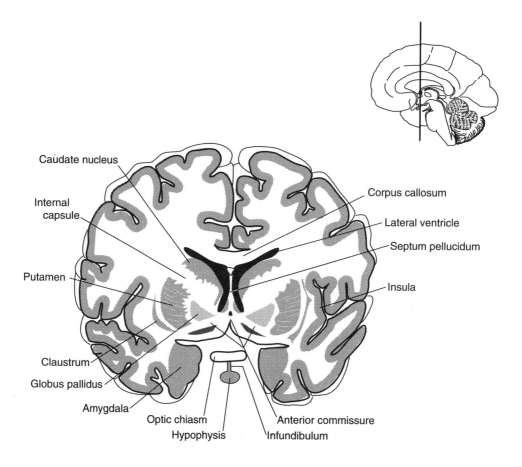

Figure 1-2.   Coronal section of the brain at the level of the anterior commissure, optic chiasm, and the amygdala. Note that the internal capsule lies between the caudate nucleus and the lentiform nucleus (globus pallidus and putamen).

L. Third ventricle

M. Fourth ventricle

III. CORONAL SECTION THROUGH THE OPTIC CHIASM (Figure 1-2). The location of the following structures should be known:

A. Amygdala

B. Anterior commissure

C. Caudate nucleus

D. Corpus callosum

E. Globus pallidus

F. Insula

G. Internal capsule

H. Lateral ventricle

I. Optic chiasm

J. Septum pellucidum

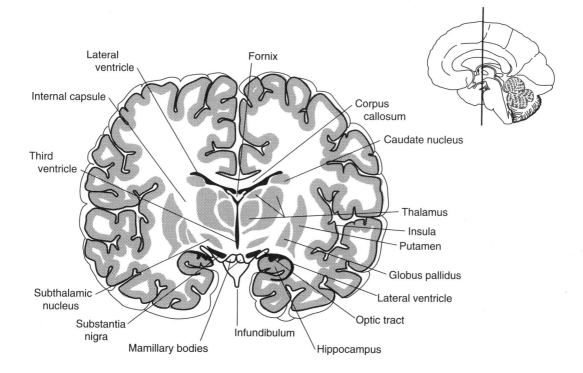

Figure 1-3. Coronal section of the brain at the level of the thalamus, mamillary bodies, and hippocampal formation. Note that the internal capsule lies between the thalamus and the lentiform nucleus.

IV. CORONAL SECTION THROUGH THE MAMILLARY BODIES (Figure 1-3). The location of the following structures should be known:

- **A.** Caudate nucleus
- **B.** Globus pallidus
- **C.** Hippocampus
- **D.** Infundibulum
- **E.** Internal capsule
- **F.** Lateral ventricle
- **G.** Mamillary body
- **H.** Optic tract
- **I.** Putamen
- **J.** Substantia nigra
- **K.** Subthalamic nucleus
- **L.** Thalamus
- **M.** Third ventricle

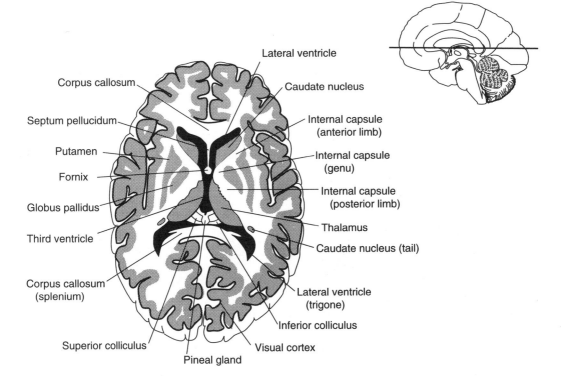

Figure 1-4. Axial section of the brain at the level of the internal capsule and the basal ganglia. Note that the internal capsule has an anterior limb, a genu, and a posterior limb. Note also that the corpus callosum is sectioned through the genu and through the splenium.

V. AXIAL IMAGE THROUGH THE THALAMUS AND INTERNAL CAPSULE (Figure 1-4).
The location of the following structures should be known:

   A. Caudate nucleus

   B. Corpus callosum

   C. Globus pallidus

   D. Internal capsule

   E. Lateral ventricle

   F. Pineal gland

   G. Putamen

   H. Superior colliculus

   I. Thalamus

   J. Third ventricle

VI. AXIAL IMAGE THROUGH THE MIDBRAIN, MAMILLARY BODIES, AND OPTIC TRACT (Figure 1-5). The location of the following structures should be known:

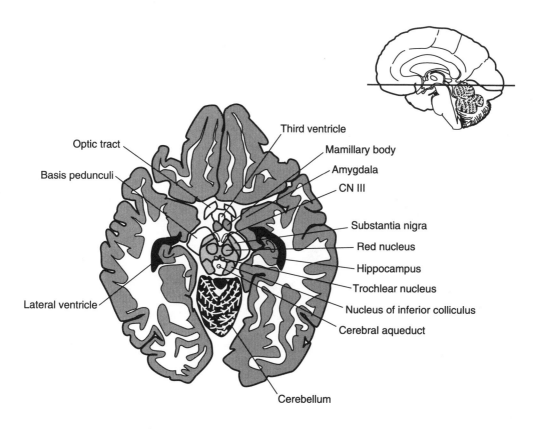

Figure 1-5. Axial section of the brain at the level of the midbrain, mamillary bodies, and the amygdala. Note that the substantia nigra separates the crus cerebri from the tegmentum of the midbrain.

A. Amygdala

B. Cerebellum

C. Cerebral aqueduct

D. Crus cerebri

E. Hippocampus

F. Inferior colliculus

G. Lateral ventricle

H. Optic tract

I. Red nucleus

J. Substantia nigra

K. Third ventricle

2

Meninges, Ventricles, and Cerebrospinal Fluid

I. MENINGES are three **connective tissue membranes** that surround the spinal cord and brain.

A. They consist of the **pia mater, arachnoid,** and **dura mater**.

1. The **pia mater** is a delicate, highly vascular layer of connective tissue that closely covers the surface of the brain and spinal cord.

2. The **arachnoid** is a delicate, nonvascular connective tissue membrane located between the dura mater and the pia mater.

3. The **dura mater** is the outer layer of meninges and consists of dense connective tissue.

B. Meningeal spaces

1. The **subarachnoid space** (Figure 2-1) lies between the pia mater and the arachnoid. It terminates at the level of the second sacral vertebra. It contains the cerebrospinal fluid (CSF).

2. Subdural space
   a. In the **cranium,** the subdural space is traversed by bridging veins.
   b. In the **spinal cord,** it is a clinically insignificant potential space.

3. Epidural space
   a. The **cranial epidural space** is a potential space; it contains the meningeal arteries and veins.
   b. The **spinal epidural space** contains fatty areolar tissue, lymphatics, and venous plexuses. The epidural space may be injected with a local anesthetic to produce a paravertebral nerve block.

C. Meningeal tumors

1. Meningiomas are benign, well-circumscribed, slow-growing tumors that account for 15% of primary intracranial tumors and are more common in women (3:2). Ninety percent of meningiomas are supratentorial.

2. Subdural and epidural hematomas
   a. Subdural hematoma is caused by laceration of the superior cerebral veins (the so-called bridging veins).
   b. Epidural hematoma is caused by laceration of the middle meningeal artery.

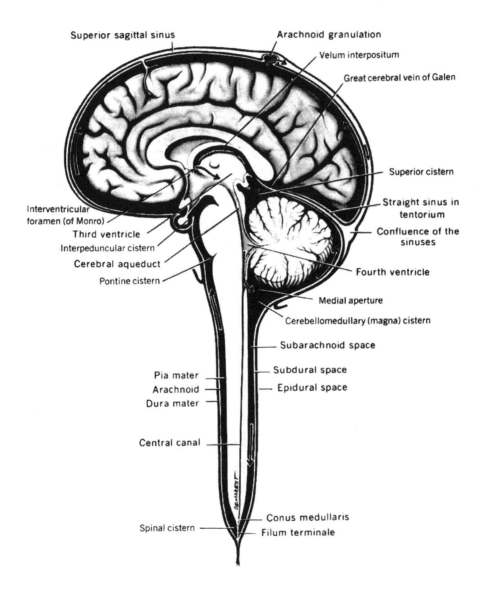

Figure 2-1.   The subarachnoid spaces and cisterns of the brain and spinal cord. Cerebrospinal fluid (CSF) is produced in the choroid plexuses of the ventricles, exits the fourth ventricle, circulates in the subarachnoid space, and enters the superior sagittal sinus via the arachnoid granulations. Note that the conus medullaris terminates at L-1. The lumbar cistern ends at S-2. (Reprinted with permission from Noback CR, Strominger NL, Demarest R: *The Human Nervous System*, 4th ed. Baltimore, Williams & Wilkins, 1991, p 68.)

D. Meningitis is inflammation of the pia–arachnoid of the brain, spinal cord, or both.

   1. Bacterial meningitis is characterized clinically by fever, headache, nuchal rigidity, and Kernig's sign. Over 70% of cases occur in children under 5 years of age. The disease may cause cranial nerve palsies and hydrocephalus.

      a. Common causes

         (1) In **newborns,** bacterial meningitis is most frequently caused by Group B streptococci (*Streptococcus agalactiae*) and *Escherichia coli.*

         (2) In **older infants and young children,** it is most frequently caused by *Haemophilus influenzae.*

         (3) In **young adults,** it is most frequently caused by *Neisseria meningitidis.*

         (4) In **older adults,** bacterial meningitis is most frequently caused by *S. pneumoniae.*

      b. CSF findings

         (1) Numerous polymorphonuclear leukocytes

         (2) Decreased glucose levels

         (3) Increased protein levels

   2. Viral meningitis is also called aseptic meningitis. It is characterized clinically by fever, headache, nuchal rigidity, and Kernig's sign.

      a. Common causes. Many viruses have been associated with viral meningitis, including mumps, echovirus, coxsackievirus, Epstein-Barr virus, and herpes simplex type 2.

      b. CSF findings

         (1) Numerous lymphocytes

         (2) Normal glucose levels

         (3) Moderately increased protein levels

II. VENTRICULAR SYSTEM

A. Choroid plexus is a specialized structure that projects into the lateral, third, and fourth ventricles of the brain. It consists of infoldings of blood vessels of the pia mater covered by modified ciliated ependymal cells. It secretes the CSF. Tight junctions of the choroid plexus cells form the blood–CSF barrier.

B. Ventricles contain CSF and choroid plexus.

   1. The two **lateral ventricles** communicate with the third ventricle via the interventricular **foramina of Monro.**

   2. The **third ventricle** is located between the medial walls of the diencephalon. It communicates with the fourth ventricle via the cerebral aqueduct.

   3. The **cerebral aqueduct** connects the third and fourth ventricles; it has no choroid plexus. Blockage of the cerebral aqueduct results in hydrocephalus.

   4. The **fourth ventricle** communicates via three outlet foramina with the subarachnoid space.

C. Hydrocephalus is dilation of the cerebral ventricles caused by blockage of the CSF pathways. It is characterized by excessive accumulation of CSF in the cerebral ventricles or subarachnoid space.

   1. Noncommunicating hydrocephalus results from obstruction within the ventricles (e.g., congenital aqueductal stenosis).

2. Communicating hydrocephalus results from blockage within the subarachnoid space (e.g., adhesions following meningitis).

3. Normal-pressure hydrocephalus results from failure of the CSF to be absorbed by the arachnoid villi; it may be secondary to post-traumatic meningeal hemorrhage. It is characterized clinically by the triad of progressive dementia, urinary incontinence, and ataxic gait.

4. Hydrocephalus ex vacuo results from a loss of cells in the caudate nucleus (e.g., in patients with Huntington's disease).

III. CEREBROSPINAL FLUID is a clear, colorless, acellular fluid that flows through the ventricles and into the subarachnoid space.

A. Function

1. The CSF **supports and protects the central nervous system (CNS)** against concussive injury.

2. It **transports hormones** and hormone-releasing factors.

3. It **removes metabolic waste products** through absorption.

B. Formation and absorption. The CSF is formed by the choroid plexus. Absorption is primarily via the arachnoid villi into the superior sagittal sinus.

C. Composition of CSF is clinically relevant.

1. The normal number of **mononuclear cells** is less than five cells per microliter.

2. Red blood cells in the CSF indicate subarachnoid hemorrhage (e.g., caused by trauma or a ruptured berry aneurysm).

3. CSF glucose levels are normally 50–75 mg/dl (66% of blood glucose). Levels are normal in patients with viral meningitis and are elevated in patients with bacterial meningitis.

4. Total protein levels are normally between 15 and 45 mg/dl in the lumbar cistern. Protein levels are elevated in patients with bacterial meningitis and are normal or slightly increased in patients with viral meningitis.

5. Normal CSF pressure in the lateral recumbent position ranges between 80 and 180 mm H_2O. Brain tumors and meningitis elevate CSF pressure.

3

Blood Supply

I. THE SPINAL CORD AND LOWER BRAIN STEM are supplied with blood through the **anterior spinal artery** (Figure 3-1).

A. The anterior spinal artery supplies the **anterior two-thirds of the spinal cord.**

B. In the **medulla,** the anterior spinal artery supplies the pyramid, medial lemniscus, and root fibers of cranial nerve (CN) XII.

II. THE INTERNAL CAROTID SYSTEM (see Figure 3-1) consists of the **internal carotid artery** and its branches.

A. The **ophthalmic artery** enters the orbit with the optic nerve (CN II). The **central artery of the retina** is a branch of the ophthalmic artery. Occlusion results in blindness.

B. The **posterior communicating artery** irrigates the hypothalamus and ventral thalamus. An **aneurysm** of this artery is the second most common aneurysm of the circle of Willis and commonly results in a **third nerve palsy.**

C. The **anterior choroidal artery** arises from the internal carotid artery and is not part of the circle of Willis. It perfuses the lateral geniculate body, the globus pallidus, and the posterior limb of the internal capsule.

D. The **anterior cerebral artery** (Figure 3-2) supplies the medial surface of the hemisphere from the frontal pole to the parieto-occipital sulcus.

    1. The anterior cerebral artery **irrigates** the **paracentral lobule,** which contains the **leg–foot area of the motor and sensory cortices.**

    2. The **anterior communicating artery** connects the two anterior cerebral arteries. It is the most common site of an **aneurysm** of the circle of Willis, which may cause a **bitemporal lower quadrantanopia.**

E. The **middle cerebral artery** (see Figure 3-2)

    1. This artery supplies the lateral convexity of the hemisphere, including:
      a. Broca's and Wernicke's speech areas
      b. The **face and arm areas** of the motor and sensory cortices
      c. Frontal eye field

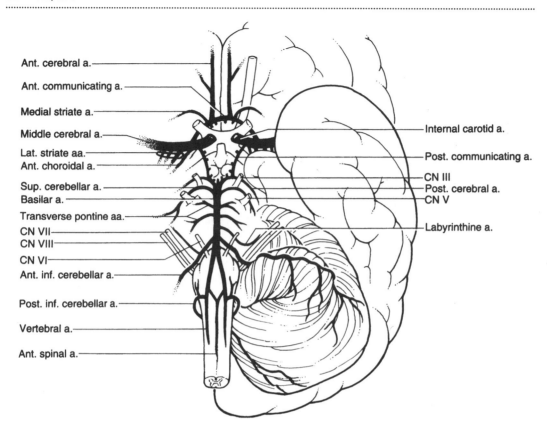

Ant. cerebral a.

Ant. communicating a.

Medial striate a.

Middle cerebral a.

Lat. striate aa.

Ant. choroidal a.

Sup. cerebellar a.

Basilar a.

Transverse pontine aa.

CN VII

CN VIII

CN VI

Ant. inf. cerebellar a.

Post. inf. cerebellar a.

Vertebral a.

Ant. spinal a.

Internal carotid a.

Post. communicating a.

CN III

Post. cerebral a.

CN V

Labyrinthine a.

Figure 3-1. Arteries of the base of the brain and brain stem, including the arterial circle of Willis.

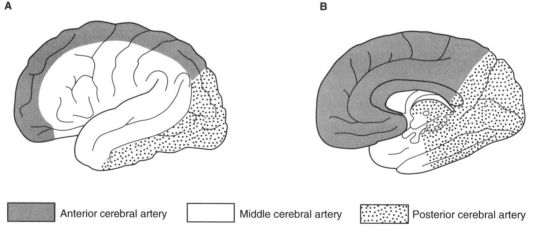

A   B

| Anterior cerebral artery | Middle cerebral artery | Posterior cerebral artery |

Figure 3-2. Cortical territories of the three cerebral arteries. (A) Lateral aspect of the hemisphere. Most of the lateral convexity is supplied by the middle cerebral artery. (B) Medial and inferior aspects of the hemisphere. The anterior cerebral artery supplies the medial surface of the hemisphere from the lamina terminalis to the cuneus. The posterior cerebral artery supplies the visual cortex and the posterior inferior surface of the temporal lobe. (Modified from Tŏndury, as presented in Sobotta J: *Atlas der Anatomie des Menschen.* Munich, Urban & Schwarzenberg, 1962, pp 137–138.)

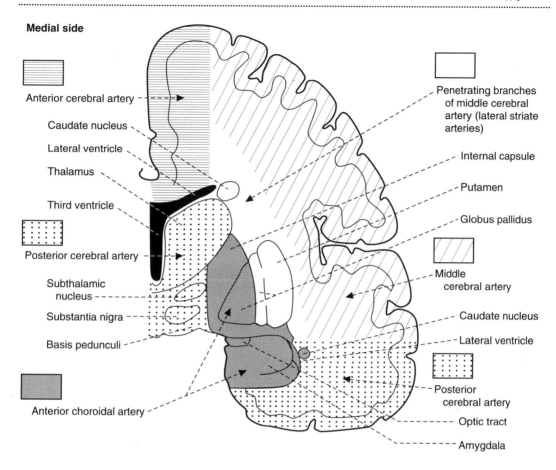

Medial side

Anterior cerebral artery

Caudate nucleus

Lateral ventricle

Thalamus

Third ventricle

Posterior cerebral artery

Subthalamic nucleus

Substantia nigra

Basis pedunculi

Anterior choroidal artery

Penetrating branches of middle cerebral artery (lateral striate arteries)

Internal capsule

Putamen

Globus pallidus

Middle cerebral artery

Caudate nucleus

Lateral ventricle

Posterior cerebral artery

Optic tract

Amygdala

Figure 3-3. Schematic drawing of a coronal section through the cerebral hemisphere at the level of the internal capsule and thalamus showing the major vascular territories.

2. The **lateral striate arteries** (Figure 3-3) are the penetrating branches of the middle cerebral artery. They are the arteries of **stroke,** and they supply the **internal capsule,** the **caudate nucleus,** the **putamen,** and the **globus pallidus.**

III. VERTEBROBASILAR SYSTEM (see Figure 3-1)

A. The **vertebral artery** is a branch of the subclavian artery. It gives rise to the **anterior spinal artery** (see I) and the **posterior inferior cerebellar artery (PICA),** which supplies the dorsolateral quadrant of the medulla, including the nucleus ambiguus (CN IX, CN X, and CN XI) and the inferior surface of the cerebellum.

B. The **basilar artery** is formed by the two vertebral arteries. It gives rise to the following arteries.

1. Paramedian branches of the **pontine arteries** supply the base of the pons, which includes the corticospinal fibers and the exiting root fibers of the abducent nerve (CN VI).

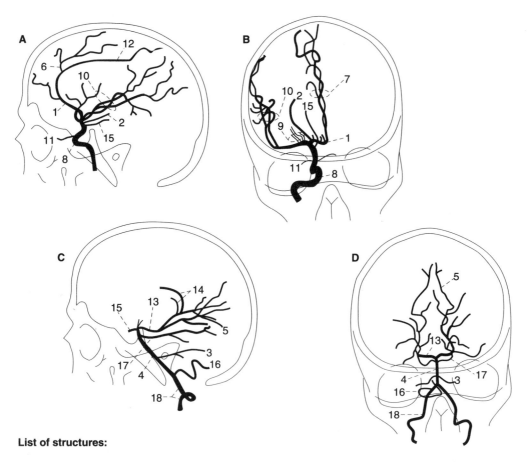

List of structures:

1. Anterior cerebral artery
2. Anterior choroidal artery
3. Anterior inferior cerebellar artery
4. Basilar artery
5. Calcarine artery (of posterior cerebral artery)
6. Callosomarginal artery (of anterior cerebral artery)
7. Callosomarginal and pericallosal arteries
   (of anterior cerebral artery)
8. Internal carotid artery
9. Lateral striate arteries (of middle cerebral artery)

10. Middle cerebral artery
11. Ophthalmic artery
12. Pericallosal artery (of anterior cerebral artery)
13. Posterior cerebral artery
14. Posterior choroidal arteries
    (of posteior cerebral artery)
15. Posterior communicating artery
16. Posterior inferior cerebellar artery
17. Superior cerebellar artery
18. Vertebral artery

Figure 3-4. (A) Carotid angiogram, lateral projection; (B) carotid angiogram, anteroposterior projection; (C) vertebral angiogram, lateral projection; (D) vertebral angiogram, anteroposterior projection.

2. The **labyrinthine artery** arises from the basilar artery in 15% of people and from the anterior inferior cerebellar artery in 85% of people.

3. The **anterior inferior cerebellar artery (AICA)** supplies the caudal lateral pontine tegmentum, including CN VII, the spinal trigeminal tract of CN V, and the inferior surface of the cerebellum.

4. The **superior cerebellar artery** supplies the dorsolateral tegmentum of the rostral pons (i.e., rostral to the motor nucleus of CN V), the superior cerebellar peduncle, and the superior surface of the cerebellum and cerebellar nuclei.

5. The **posterior cerebral artery** (see Figures 3-1, 3-2, and 3-3) is connected to the carotid artery via the posterior communicating artery. It provides the **major blood supply to the midbrain**. It also supplies the thalamus and the lateral and medial geniculate bodies, as well as the occipital lobe with visual cortex and the inferior surface of the temporal lobe (including the hippocampal formation). **Occlusion** of this artery results in a **contralateral hemianopia with macular sparing**.

IV. BLOOD SUPPLY OF THE INTERNAL CAPSULE comes primarily from the **lateral striate arteries** of the middle cerebral artery and the **anterior choroidal artery**.

V. VEINS OF THE BRAIN

   A. The **superior cerebral veins (bridging veins)** drain into the superior sagittal sinus. Laceration results in a **subdural hematoma**.

   B. The **great cerebral vein of Galen** drains the deep cerebral veins into the **straight sinus**.

VI. VENOUS DURAL SINUSES

   A. The **superior sagittal sinus** receives the bridging veins, and via the arachnoid villi, the cerebrospinal fluid (CSF).

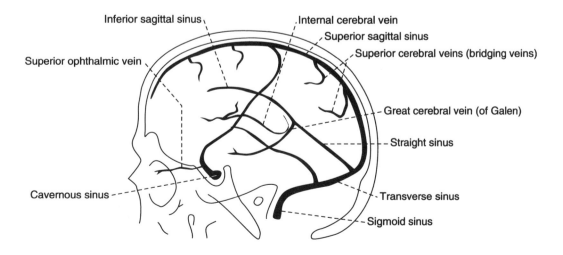

Figure 3-5.   Carotid angiogram, venous phase, lateral projection showing cerebral veins and venous sinuses.

   B. The **cavernous sinus** contains CN III, CN IV, CN V-1 and V-2, CN VI, and postganglionic sympathetic fibers. It contains the siphon of the internal carotid artery.

VII. ANGIOGRAPHY

   A. **Carotid angiography.** Figures 3-4A and B show the internal carotid artery, the anterior cerebral artery, and the middle cerebral artery.

   B. **Vertebral angiography.** Figures 3-4C and D show the vertebral artery, the PICA and AICA, the basilar artery, the superior cerebellar artery, and the posterior cerebral artery.

   C. **Veins and dural sinuses.** Figure 3-5 shows the internal cerebral vein, the superior cerebral veins, the great cerebral vein, the superior ophthalmic vein, and the major dural sinuses.

VIII. MIDDLE MENINGEAL ARTERY, a branch of the **maxillary artery,** enters the cranium via the **foramen spinosum**. It supplies most of the dura including its calvarial portion. Laceration results in **epidural hemorrhage** (hematoma).

4

Development of the Nervous System

I. **THE NEURAL TUBE** (Figure 4-1) gives rise to the **central nervous system (CNS)**—that is, the brain and spinal cord.

    A. The **brain stem** and spinal cord have:

        1. An **alar plate** that gives rise to **sensory neurons**

        2. A **basal plate** that gives rise to **motor neurons** (Figure 4-2)

    B. The neural tube gives rise to **three primary vesicles,** which develop into **five secondary vesicles** (Figure 4-3).

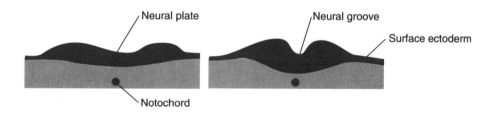

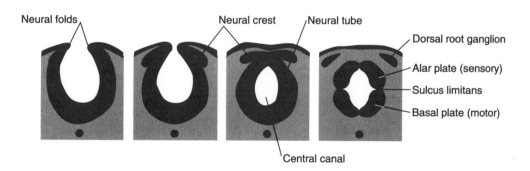

Figure 4-1. Development of the neural tube and neural crest. The alar plate gives rise to sensory neurons; the basal plate gives rise to motor neurons. The neural crest gives rise to the peripheral nervous system (PNS).

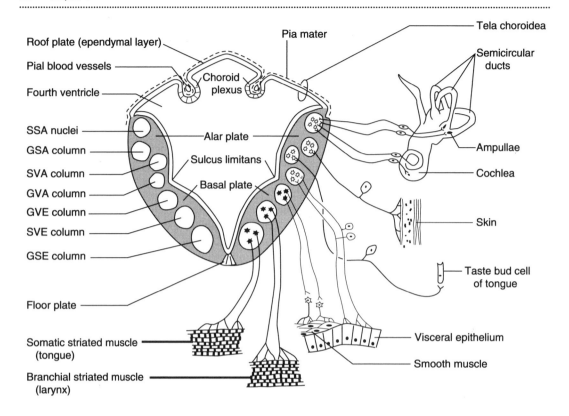

Figure 4-2. Schematic drawing of the brain stem showing the cell columns derived from the alar and basal plates. The seven cranial nerve modalities are shown. GSA = general somatic afferent; GSE = general somatic efferent; GVA = general visceral afferent; GVE = general visceral efferent; SSA = special somatic afferent; SVA = special visceral afferent; SVE = special visceral efferent. (Adapted with permission from Patten BM: *Human Embryology*, 3rd ed. New York, The Blakiston Division, McGraw-Hill, 1969, p 298.)

 C. Alpha-fetoprotein (AFP) is found in the amniotic fluid and maternal serum. It is an indicator of neural tube defects (e.g., spina bifida, anencephaly). Reduced levels of AFP are found in mothers of fetuses with Down syndrome.

II. THE NEURAL CREST (see Figure 4-1) gives rise to:

 A. The **peripheral nervous system (PNS)**—that is, the peripheral nerves and the sensory and autonomic ganglia.

 B. The following cells:

  1. Pseudounipolar ganglion cells of spinal and cranial nerve ganglia

  2. Schwann cells (elaborate the myelin sheath)

  3. Multipolar ganglion cells of autonomic ganglia

  4. Leptomeninges (pia-arachnoid)

  5. Chromaffin cells of the suprarenal medulla (elaborate epinephrine)

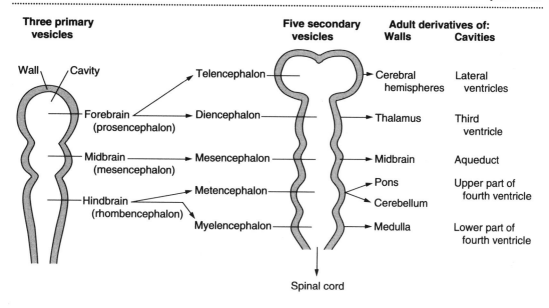

Figure 4-3. Diagrammatic sketches of the brain vesicles indicating the adult derivatives of their walls and cavities. (Reprinted with permission from Moore KL: *The Developing Human: Clinically Oriented Embryology,* 4th ed. Philadelphia, WB Saunders, 1988, p 380.)

6. **Pigment cells** (melanocytes)

7. **Odontoblasts** (elaborate predentin)

III. ANTERIOR NEUROPORE. The closure of the anterior neuropore gives rise to the lamina terminalis. **Failure to close results in anencephaly,** which is failure of the brain to develop.

IV. POSTERIOR NEUROPORE. Failure to close results in spina bifida (Figure 4-4).

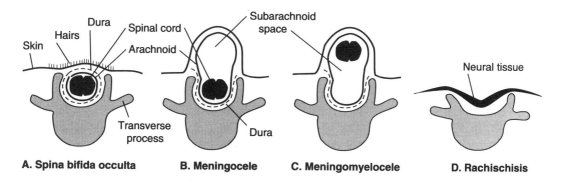

Figure 4-4. Schematic drawings illustrating the various types of spina bifida. (Reprinted with permission from Sadler TW: *Langman's Medical Embryology,* 6th ed. Baltimore, Williams & Wilkins, 1990, p 363.)

V. MICROGLIA arise from monocytes.

VI. MYELINATION commences in the fourth month of gestation. Myelination of the cortico-spinal tracts is not completed until the end of the second postnatal year, at which time the tracts become functional. Myelination in the cerebral association cortex continues into the third decade.

  A. Myelination of the CNS is accomplished by oligodendrocytes, which are not found in the retina.

  B. Myelination of the PNS is accomplished by Schwann cells.

VII. POSITIONAL CHANGES OF THE SPINAL CORD

  A. In the **newborn,** the conus medullaris ends at the third lumbar vertebra (L-3).

  B. In the **adult,** the conus medullaris ends at L-1.

VIII. OPTIC NERVE AND CHIASMA are derived from the diencephalon. The optic nerve fibers occupy the **choroid fissure**. Failure of this fissure to close results in **coloboma iridis**.

IX. HYPOPHYSIS (pituitary gland) is derived from two embryologic substrata (Figure 4-5).

  A. Adenohypophysis is derived from an ectodermal diverticulum of the primitive mouth cavity (stomodeum), which is also called **Rathke's pouch**. Remnants of Rathke's pouch may give rise to a congenital cystic tumor, a **craniopharyngioma**.

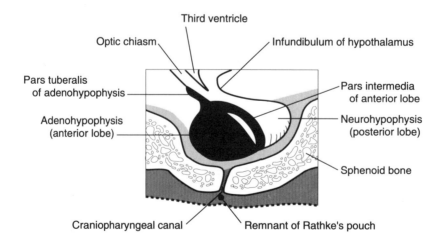

Figure 4-5.   Midsagittal section through the hypophysis and sella turcica. The adenohypophysis, including the pars tuberalis and the pars intermedia, is derived from Rathke's pouch (oroectoderm). The neurohypophysis arises from the infundibulum of the hypothalamus (neuroectoderm).

B. **Neurohypophysis** develops from a ventral evagination of the hypothalamus (neuroectoderm of the neural tube).

X. CONGENITAL MALFORMATIONS OF THE CNS

A. **Anencephaly (meroanencephaly)** results from failure of the anterior neuropore to close; the brain fails to develop; frequency 1:1000.

B. **Spina bifida** results from failure of the posterior neuropore to form; usually occurs in the sacrolumbar region; frequency of **spina bifida occulta** is 10%.

C. **Cranium bifidum** results from a defect in the occipital bone through which meninges, cerebellar tissue, and fourth ventricle may herniate.

D. **Arnold-Chiari syndrome** is a cerebellomedullary malformation in which the caudal vermis, cerebellar tonsils, and medulla herniate through the foramen magnum, resulting in a communicating hydrocephalus; frequency 1:1000.

E. **Dandy-Walker syndrome** is a hydrocephalus resulting from failure of the foramina of Luschka and Magendie to open; associated with an occipital meningocele and agenesis of the cerebellar vermis and splenium of the corpus callosum.

F. **Hydrocephalus** is most commonly caused by stenosis of the cerebral aqueduct during development. Excessive CSF accumulates in the ventricles and subarachnoid space; may result from maternal infection (cytomegalovirus and toxoplasmosis); frequency 1:1000.

G. **Fetal alcohol syndrome** is the most common cause of mental retardation. It includes microcephaly and congenital heart disease; holoprosencephaly is the most severe manifestation.

5

Neurohistology

I. NEURONS may be classified by the number of processes (Figure 5-1).

    A. Pseudounipolar neurons are located in the spinal dorsal root ganglia and in the sensory ganglia of cranial nerves (CN) V, VII, IX, and X.

    B. Bipolar neurons are found in the cochlear and vestibular ganglia of CN VIII, in the olfactory nerve (CN I), and in the retina.

    C. Multipolar neurons are the largest population of nerve cells in the nervous system. These include motor neurons, neurons of the autonomic nervous system, interneurons, pyramidal cells of the cerebral cortex, and Purkinje's cells of the cerebellar cortex.

II. NISSL SUBSTANCE is characteristic of neurons and consists of rosettes of polysomes and rough endoplasmic reticulum and, therefore, has a role in protein synthesis. Nissl substance is found in the **nerve cell body (perikaryon)** and **dendrites,** not in the axon hillock or in the axon.

III. AXONAL TRANSPORT mediates the intracellular distribution of secretory proteins, organelles, and cytoskeletal elements. It is inhibited by colchicine, which depolymerizes microtubules.

    A. Fast anterograde axonal transport is responsible for transporting all newly synthesized membranous organelles (vesicles) and precursors of neurotransmitters at the rate of 200–400 mm/day. It is mediated by neurotubules and **kinesin** (fast transport is neurotubule-dependent).

    B. Slow anterograde transport is responsible for transporting fibrillar cytoskeletal and protoplasmic elements at the rate of 1–5 mm/day.

    C. Fast retrograde transport returns used materials from the axon terminal to the cell body for degradation and recycling at a rate of 100–200 mm/day. It transports **nerve growth factor, neurotropic viruses,** and toxins (e.g., **herpes simplex, rabies, poliovirus, tetanus toxin**). It is mediated by neurotubules and **dynein.**

IV. WALLERIAN DEGENERATION is anterograde degeneration characterized by the disappearance of axons and myelin sheaths and secondary proliferation of Schwann cells. It occurs in the central nervous system (CNS) and the peripheral nervous system (PNS).

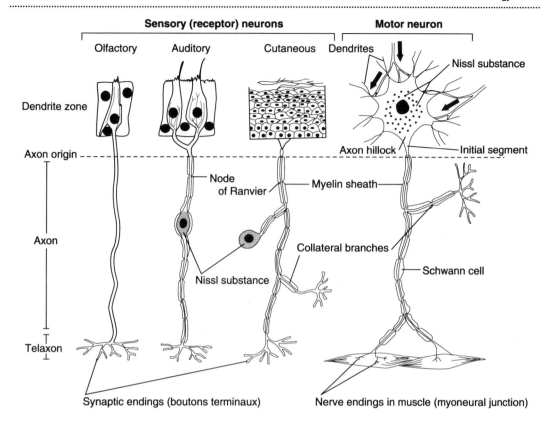

Figure 5-1.   Types of nerve cells. *Olfactory* neurons are bipolar and unmyelinated. *Auditory* neurons are bipolar and myelinated. *Dorsal root ganglion* cells (cutaneous) are pseudounipolar and myelinated. *Motor* neurons are multipolar and myelinated. *Arrows* indicate input via axons of other neurons. Nerve cells are characterized by the presence of Nissl substance, rough endoplasmic reticulum. (Modified with permission from Carpenter MB, Sutin J: *Human Neuroanatomy.* Baltimore, Williams & Wilkins, 1983, p 92.)

   V. CHROMATOLYSIS is the result of retrograde degeneration in the neurons of the CNS and PNS. There is a loss of Nissl substance after axotomy.

VI. REGENERATION OF NERVE CELLS

   A. CNS. Effective regeneration does not occur in the CNS. For example, there is no regeneration of the optic nerve, which is a tract of the diencephalon. There are no basement membranes or endoneural investments surrounding the axons of the CNS.

   B. PNS. Regeneration does occur in the PNS. The proximal tip of a severed axon grows into the endoneural tube, which consists of Schwann cell basement membrane and endoneurium. The axon sprout grows at the rate of 3 mm/day.

VII. GLIAL CELLS are the non-neural cells of the nervous system.

   A. Macroglia consists of **astrocytes and oligodendrocytes**.

    1. Astrocytes perform the following functions:

      a. They project foot processes that envelop the basement membrane of capillaries, neurons, and synapses.

      b. They form the external and internal glial-limiting membranes of the CNS.

      c. They play a role in the metabolism of certain neurotransmitters (e.g., GABA, serotonin, glutamate).

      d. They buffer the potassium concentration of the extracellular space.

      e. They form glial scars in damaged areas of the brain (i.e., astrogliosis).

      f. They contain glial fibrillary acidic protein (GFAP), which is a marker for astrocytes.

    2. Oligodendrocytes are the myelin-forming cells of the CNS. One oligodendrocyte can myelinate up to 30 axons.

B. Microglia arise from monocytes and function as the scavenger cells (phagocytes) of the CNS.

C. Ependymal cells are ciliated cells that line the central canal and the ventricles of the brain. They also line the luminal surface of the choroid plexus and **produce cerebrospinal fluid (CSF).**

D. Schwann cells are derived from the neural crest. They are the myelin-forming cells of the PNS; one Schwann cell can myelinate only one internode. Schwann cells invest all myelinated and unmyelinated axons of the PNS and are separated from each other by the **nodes of Ranvier.**

VIII. THE BLOOD–BRAIN BARRIER consists of the tight junctions of nonfenestrated endothelial cells; some authorities include the astrocytic foot processes. **Infarction of brain tissue** destroys the tight junctions of endothelial cells and results in **vasogenic edema,** which is an infiltrate of plasma into the extracellular space.

IX. PIGMENTS AND INCLUSIONS

A. Lipofuscin granules are pigmented cytoplasmic inclusions that commonly accumulate with aging. They are considered to be residual bodies derived from lysosomes.

B. Melanin (neuromelanin) is blackish intracytoplasmic pigment found in the substantia nigra and the locus coeruleus. It disappears from nigral neurons in patients with Parkinson's disease.

C. Lewy bodies are neuronal inclusions that are characteristic of Parkinson's disease.

D. Negri bodies are intracytoplasmic inclusions that are pathognomonic of rabies. They are found in the pyramidal cells of the hippocampus and in the Purkinje cells of the cerebellum.

E. Hirano bodies are intraneuronal, eosinophilic rod-like inclusions found in the hippocampus of patients with Alzheimer's disease.

F. Neurofibrillary tangles consist of intracytoplasmic degenerated neurofilaments and are seen in patients with Alzheimer's disease.

X. CLASSIFICATION OF NERVE FIBERS is given in Table 5-1.

Table 5–1
Classification of Nerve Fibers

Fibers	Diameter (μm)*	Conduction Velocity (m/sec)	Function
Sensory axons			
Ia (A-α)	12–20	70–120	Proprioception, muscle spindles
Ib (A-α)	12–20	70–120	Proprioception, Golgi tendon organs
II (A-β)	5–12	30–70	Touch, pressure, and vibration
III (A-δ)	2–5	12–30	Touch, pressure, fast pain, and temperature
IV (C)	0.5–1	0.5–2	Slow pain and temperature, unmyelinated fibers
Motor axons			
Alpha (A-α)	12–20	15–120	Alpha motor neurons of ventral horn (innervate extrafusal muscle fibers)
Gamma (A-γ)	2–10	10–45	Gamma motor neurons of ventral horn (innervate intrafusal muscle fibers)
Preganglionic autonomic fibers (B)	< 3	3–15	Myelinated preganglionic autonomic fibers
Postganglionic autonomic fibers (C)	1	2	Unmyelinated postganglionic autonomic fibers

*Myelin sheath included if present.

6

Spinal Cord

I. GRAY AND WHITE COMMUNICATING RAMI (Figure 6-1)

A. **Gray communicating rami** contain unmyelinated postganglionic sympathetic fibers and are found at all spinal cord levels.

B. **White communicating rami** contain myelinated preganglionic sympathetic fibers and are found from T-1 to L-3 (the extent of the lateral horn and the intermediolateral cell column).

II. TERMINATION OF CONUS MEDULLARIS (see Figure 2-1) occurs in the newborn at the level of the body of the third lumbar vertebra (L-3) and in the adult at the level of the lower border of the first lumbar vertebra (L-1).

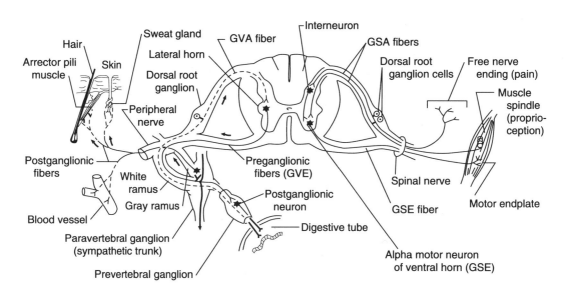

Figure 6-1. Diagram of the four functional components of the thoracic spinal nerve: general visceral afferent (GVA), general somatic afferent (GSA), general somatic efferent (GSE), and general visceral efferent (GVE). Proprioceptive, cutaneous, and visceral reflex arcs are shown. The muscle stretch (myotatic) reflex includes the muscle spindle, GSA dorsal root ganglion cell, GSE ventral horn motor neuron, and skeletal muscle.

III. LOCATION OF MAJOR MOTOR AND SENSORY NUCLEI OF THE SPINAL CORD

A. Ciliospinal center of Budge from C-8 to T-2, which mediates the sympathetic innervation of the eye

B. Intermediolateral cell column from C-8 to L-3, which mediates the entire sympathetic innervation of the body

C. Nucleus dorsalis of Clarke from C-8 to L-3, which gives rise to the dorsal spinocerebellar tract

D. Parasympathetic nucleus from S-2 to S-4

E. Spinal accessory nucleus from C-1 to C-6

F. Phrenic nucleus from C-3 to C-6

IV. CAUDA EQUINA.
Motor and sensory roots (L-2 to Co) that are found in the subarachnoid space below the conus medullaris form the cauda equina. They exit the vertebral canal via the lumbar intervertebral and sacral foramina.

V. MYOTATIC REFLEX
(see Figure 6-1) is a monosynaptic and ipsilateral **muscle stretch reflex (MSR)**. Like all reflexes, the myotatic reflex has an afferent and an efferent limb. **Interruption of either limb** results in **areflexia**.

A. The **afferent limb** includes a muscle spindle (receptor) and a dorsal root ganglion neuron and its Ia fiber.

B. The **efferent limb** includes a ventral horn motor neuron that innervates striated muscle (effector).

C. The four most commonly tested MSRs are listed in Table 6-1.

Table 6–1
Four Most Commonly Tested Muscle Stretch Reflexes (MSRs)

MSR	Cord Segment	Muscle
Ankle jerk	S-1	Gastrocnemius
Knee jerk	L-2–L-4	Quadriceps
Biceps jerk	C-5 and C-6	Biceps
Triceps jerk	C-7 and C-8	Triceps

7

Tracts of the Spinal Cord

I. **INTRODUCTION.** Figure 7-1 shows the ascending and descending tracts of the spinal cord. Four of the major tracts are covered in this chapter.

II. **DORSAL COLUMN–MEDIAL LEMNISCUS PATHWAY** (Figure 7-2; see also Figure 8-1)

    A. **Function.** The dorsal column–medial lemniscus pathway mediates tactile discrimination, vibration sensation, form recognition, and joint and muscle sensation (conscious proprioception).

    B. **Receptors** include Pacini's and Meissner's tactile corpuscles, joint receptors, muscle spindles, and Golgi tendon organs.

    C. **First-order neurons** are located in dorsal root ganglia at all levels. They project axons to the spinal cord via the medial root entry zone. First-order neurons give rise to:

        1. The gracile fasciculus from the lower extremity

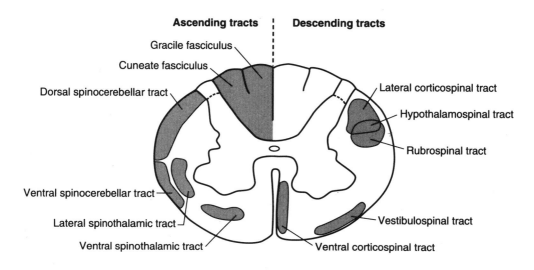

Figure 7-1. Schematic diagram of the major ascending and descending pathways of the spinal cord. Ascending sensory tracts are shown on the *left*; descending motor tracts are shown on the *right*.

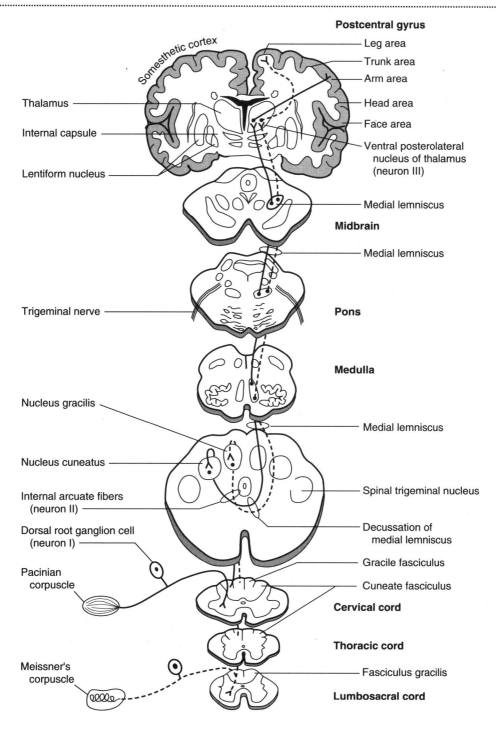

Figure 7-2. Schematic diagram of the dorsal column–medial lemniscus pathway. Impulses conducted by this pathway mediate discriminatory tactile sense (touch, vibration, pressure) and kinesthetic sense (position, movement). The dorsal column system mediates conscious proprioception. (Adapted with permission from Carpenter MB, Sutin J: *Human Neuroanatomy.* Baltimore, Williams & Wilkins, 1983, p 266.)

    2. The cuneate fasciculus from the upper extremity

    3. The collaterals for spinal reflexes (e.g., myotatic reflex)

    4. The axons that ascend in the dorsal columns and terminate in the gracile and cuneate nuclei of the caudal medulla

D. Second-order neurons are located in the gracile and cuneate nuclei of the caudal medulla. They give rise to axons and internal arcuate fibers that decussate and form a compact fiber bundle called the medial lemniscus. The medial lemniscus ascends through the contralateral brain stem to terminate in the ventral posterolateral (VPL) nucleus of the thalamus.

E. Third-order neurons are located in the VPL nucleus of the thalamus. They project via the posterior limb of the internal capsule to the postcentral gyrus, which is the primary somatosensory cortex (Brodmann's areas 3, 1, and 2).

F. Transection of the dorsal column–medial lemniscus tract

    1. Above the sensory decussation there is contralateral loss of dorsal column modalities.

    2. In the spinal cord there is ipsilateral loss of dorsal column modalities.

III. LATERAL SPINOTHALAMIC TRACT (Figure 7-3; see also Figure 8-1)

A. Function. The lateral spinothalamic tract mediates pain and temperature sensation.

B. Receptors are free nerve endings. The lateral spinothalamic tract receives input from fast- and slow-conducting pain fibers (i.e., A-δ and C, respectively).

C. First-order neurons are found in dorsal root ganglia at all levels. They project axons to the spinal cord via the dorsolateral tract of Lissauer (lateral root entry zone) to second-order neurons.

D. Second-order neurons are found in the dorsal horn. They give rise to axons that decussate in the **ventral white commissure** and ascend in the contralateral lateral funiculus. Their axons terminate in the VPL nucleus of the thalamus.

E. Third-order neurons are found in the VPL nucleus of the thalamus. They project via the posterior limb of the internal capsule to the primary somatosensory cortex (Brodmann's areas 3, 1, and 2).

F. Transection of the lateral spinothalamic tract results in a contralateral loss of pain and temperature below the lesion.

IV. LATERAL CORTICOSPINAL TRACT (Figure 7-4; see also Figure 8-1)

A. Function. The lateral corticospinal tract mediates voluntary skilled motor activity, primarily of the upper limbs. It is not fully myelinated until the end of the second year (Babinski's sign).

B. Fiber caliber. Approximately 90% of the fibers lie between 1 and 4 μm, and 4% lie above 20 μm (from the giant cells of Betz).

C. Origin and termination

    1. Origin. The lateral corticospinal tract arises from layer V of the cerebral cortex from three cortical areas in equal aliquots:
        a. The **premotor cortex** (Brodmann's area 6)

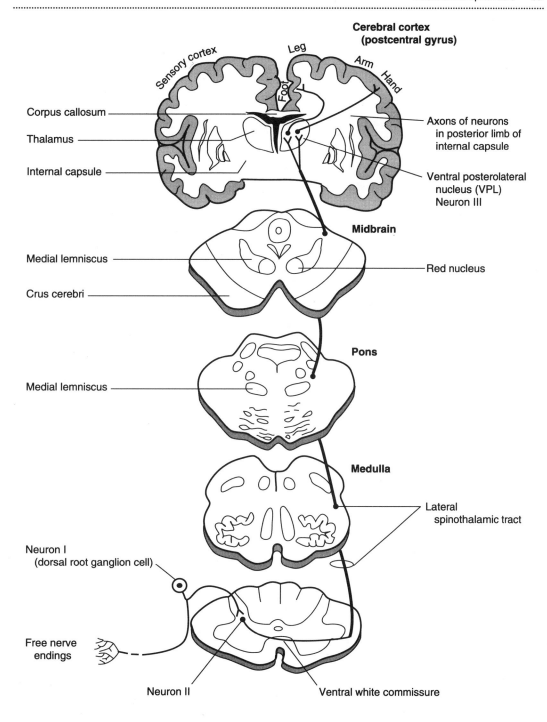

Figure 7-3.   Schematic diagram of the lateral spinothalamic tract. Impulses conducted by this tract mediate pain and thermal sense. Numerous collaterals are distributed to the brain stem reticular formation. (Reprinted with permission from Carpenter MB, Sutin J: *Human Neuroanatomy*. Baltimore, Williams & Wilkins, 1983, p 274.)

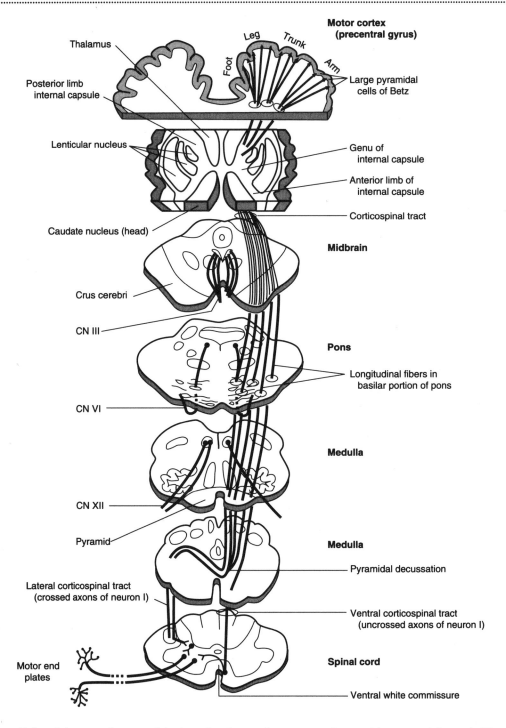

Figure 7-4. Schematic diagram of the lateral and ventral corticospinal tracts (the pyramidal tracts). These major descending motor pathways mediate volitional motor activity. The cells of origin are located in the premotor, the motor, and the sensory cortices. (Reprinted with permission from Carpenter MB, Sutin J: *Human Neuroanatomy.* Baltimore, Williams & Wilkins, 1983, p 285.)

    b. The **primary motor cortex** (Brodmann's area 4)

    c. The **primary sensory cortex** (Brodmann's areas 3, 1, and 2)

    d. Note. The arm and face areas of the motor homunculus arise from the lateral convexity; the foot area arises from the paracentral lobule.

  2. Termination. The lateral corticospinal tract terminates contralaterally, via interneurons, on ventral horn motor neurons.

D. Course of lateral corticospinal tract

  1. Telencephalon. The lateral corticospinal tract runs in the posterior limb of the internal capsule in the telencephalon.

  2. Midbrain. The lateral corticospinal tract runs in the middle three-fifths of the crus cerebri in the midbrain.

  3. Pons. The lateral corticospinal tract runs in the base of the pons.

  4. Medulla. The lateral corticospinal tract runs in the medullary pyramids (85% to 90% of the corticospinal fibers decussate in pyramidal decussation as the lateral corticospinal tract; the remaining 10% to 15% continue as the anterior corticospinal tract).

  5. Spinal cord. The lateral corticospinal tract runs in the dorsal quadrant of the lateral funiculus.

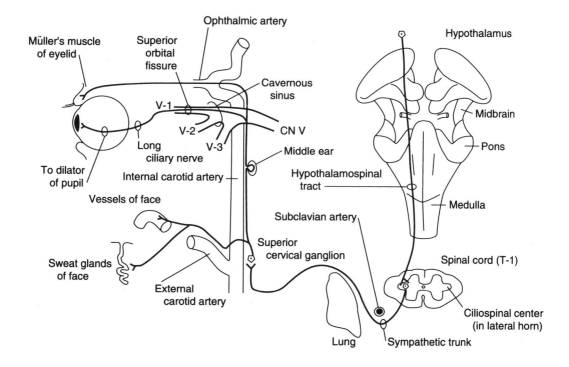

Figure 7-5. Oculosympathetic pathway. Hypothalamic fibers project to the ipsilateral ciliospinal center of the intermediolateral cell column at T-1. The ciliospinal center projects preganglionic sympathetic fibers to the superior cervical ganglion (SCG). The SCG projects perivascular postganglionic sympathetic fibers via the tympanic cavity, cavernous sinus, and superior orbital fissure to the dilator muscle of the iris. Interruption of this pathway at any level results in Horner's syndrome.

    E. Transection of lateral corticospinal tract

        1. Above the motor decussation, transection results in contralateral spastic paresis and Babinski's sign.

        2. In the spinal cord, transection results in ipsilateral spastic paresis and Babinski's sign (upgoing toe).

V. HYPOTHALAMOSPINAL TRACT (Figure 7-5)

    A. Anatomic location. The hypothalamospinal tract projects without interruption from the hypothalamus to the ciliospinal center of the intermediolateral cell column at T-1 to T-2. It is found in the spinal cord at T-1 or above in the dorsolateral quadrant of the lateral funiculus. It is also found in the lateral tegmentum of the medulla, pons, and midbrain.

    B. Clinical. Interruption of this tract at any level results in Horner's syndrome (miosis, ptosis, hemianhidrosis, and apparent enophthalmos). The signs are always ipsilateral.

8

s of the Spinal Cord

NEURONS AND CORTICOSPINAL TRACTS (Figures 8-1

UMN) lesions are caused by transection of the corticospinal
he cortical cells of origin. They result in **spastic paresis** with
i's sign).

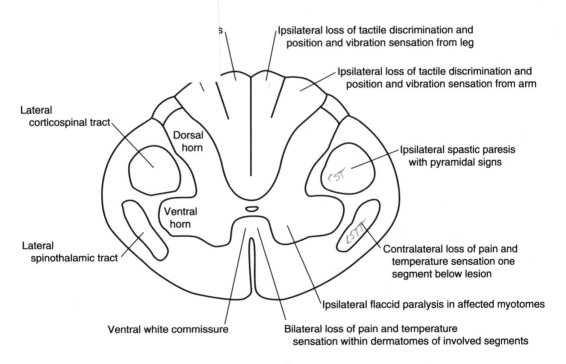

Figure 8-1. Transverse section of the cervical spinal cord showing, on the *left side*, the clinically important ascending and descending pathways. Clinical deficits resulting from the interruption of these pathways are shown on the *right side*. Destructive lesions of the dorsal horns result in anesthesia and areflexia. Destructive lesions of the ventral horns result in lower motor neuron lesions and areflexia. Destruction of the ventral white commissure interrupts the central transmission of pain and temperature impulses bilaterally via the lateral spinothalamic tracts.

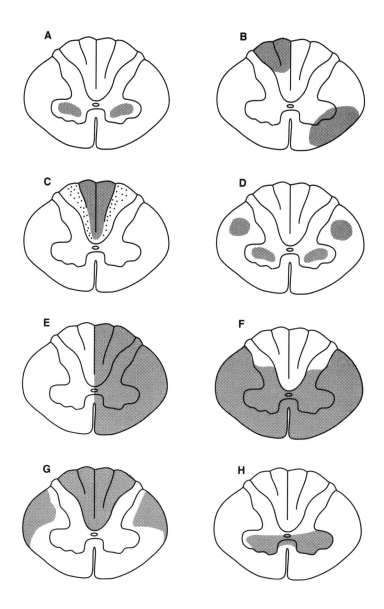

Figure 8-2. Classic lesions of the spinal cord: (A) poliomyelitis and progressive infantile muscular atrophy (Werdnig-Hoffmann disease); (B) multiple sclerosis; (C) dorsal column disease (tabes dorsalis); (D) amyotrophic lateral sclerosis (ALS); (E) hemisection of the spinal cord (Brown-Séquard syndrome); (F) complete ventral artery occlusion of the spinal cord; (G) subacute combined degeneration (vitamin B_{12} neuropathy); (H) syringomyelia.

B. **Lower motor neuron (LMN) lesions** are caused by damage to motor neurons. They result in **flaccid paralysis,** areflexia, atrophy, fasciculations, and fibrillations. **Poliomyelitis or Werdnig-Hoffmann disease** (see Figure 8-2A) results from damage to motor neurons.

C. **Combined UMN and LMN disease.** An example of a combined UMN and LMN disease is **amyotrophic lateral sclerosis** (i.e., **ALS; Lou Gehrig's disease**) [see Figure 8-2D]. ALS is caused by damage to the corticospinal tracts, with pyramidal signs, and by damage to LMNs, with LMN symptoms. There are no sensory deficits in patients with ALS.

II. SENSORY PATHWAY LESIONS.

An example of a condition caused by these lesions is **dorsal column disease (tabes dorsalis)** [see Figure 8-2C]. This disease is seen in patients with neurosyphilis and is characterized by a loss of tactile discrimination and position and vibration sensation. Irritative involvement of the dorsal roots results in pain and paresthesias. Patients have a Romberg sign (dorsal column ataxia).

III. COMBINED MOTOR AND SENSORY LESIONS

A. **Spinal cord hemisection (Brown-Séquard syndrome)** [see Figure 8-2E] is caused by damage to the following structures:

1. **Dorsal columns [gracile (leg) and cuneate (arm) fasciculi],** which results in ipsilateral loss of tactile discrimination, position sensation, and vibration sensation

2. **Lateral corticospinal tract,** which results in ipsilateral spastic paresis with pyramidal signs below the lesion

3. **Lateral spinothalamic tract,** which results in contralateral loss of pain and temperature sensation one segment below the lesion

4. **Hypothalamospinal tract at T-1 and above,** which results in ipsilateral Horner's syndrome (miosis, ptosis, hemianhidrosis, and apparent enophthalmos)

5. **Ventral (anterior) horn,** which results in ipsilateral flaccid paralysis of innervated muscles

B. **Ventral spinal artery occlusion** (see Figure 8-2F) causes infarction of the anterior two-thirds of the spinal cord, but spares the dorsal columns and dorsal horns. It results in damage to the following structures:

1. **Lateral corticospinal tracts,** which results in bilateral spastic paresis with pyramidal signs below the lesion

2. **Lateral spinothalamic tracts,** which results in bilateral loss of pain and temperature sensation below the lesion

3. **Hypothalamospinal tract at T-2 and above,** which results in bilateral Horner's syndrome

4. **Ventral (anterior) horns,** which results in bilateral flaccid paralysis of innervated muscles

5. **Corticospinal tracts to sacral parasympathetic centers at S-2 to S-4,** which results in bilateral damage and loss of voluntary bladder and bowel control

C. Subacute combined degeneration (vitamin B$_{12}$ neuropathy) [see Figure 8-2G] is caused by pernicious anemia (megaloblastic anemia). It results from damage to the following structures:

1. **Dorsal columns (gracile and cuneate fasciculi),** which results in bilateral loss of tactile discrimination and position and vibration sensation

2. **Lateral corticospinal tracts,** which results in bilateral spastic paresis with pyramidal signs

3. **Spinocerebellar tracts,** which results in bilateral arm and leg dystaxia

D. Syringomyelia (see Figure 8-2H) is a central cavitation of the cervical cord of unknown etiology. It results in damage to the following structures:

1. **Ventral white commissure.** Damage to decussating lateral spinothalamic axons causes a bilateral loss of pain and temperature sensation.

2. **Ventral horns.** LMN lesions result in a flaccid paralysis of the intrinsic muscles of the hands.

E. **Friedreich's ataxia** has the same spinal cord pathology and symptomatology as subacute combined degeneration.

F. **Multiple sclerosis** (see Figure 8-2B). Plaques involve mostly the white matter of cervical segments of the spinal cord. The lesions are random and asymmetric.

IV. PERIPHERAL NERVOUS SYSTEM (PNS) LESIONS. An example of a PNS lesion is **Guillain-Barré syndrome (acute idiopathic polyneuritis),** which is also called postinfectious polyneuritis. It affects primarily the motor fibers of ventral roots and peripheral nerves and produces LMN symptoms (i.e., muscle weakness, flaccid paralysis, areflexia).

A. **Facial diplegia occurs in 50% of cases.**

B. To a lesser degree, sensory fibers are affected, resulting in paresthesias.

C. The protein level in the cerebrospinal fluid (CSF) is elevated but with normal CSF cell count (albuminocytological dissociation).

V. INTERVERTEBRAL DISK HERNIATION appears in 90% of cases at the L-4 to L-5 or L-5 to S-1 interspaces. In 10% of cases, it appears at the C-5 to C-6 or C-6 to C-7 interspaces.

A. Intervertebral disk herniation consists of prolapse or herniation of the **nucleus pulposus through the defective anulus fibrosus into the vertebral canal.**

B. The nucleus pulposus **impinges on spinal roots,** resulting in spinal root symptoms, which include paresthesias, pain, sensory loss, hyporeflexia, and muscle weakness.

9

Brain Stem

I. **OVERVIEW.** The brain stem includes the **medulla, pons,** and **midbrain.** It extends from the pyramidal decussation to the posterior commissure. The brain stem receives its blood supply from the vertebrobasilar system. It contains cranial nerves (CN) III to XII (except the spinal part of CN XI). Figures 9-1 and 9-2 show the surface anatomy of the brain stem.

II. **CROSS SECTION THROUGH THE MEDULLA** (Figure 9-3)

    A. Medial structures

        1. Hypoglossal nucleus of CN XII

        2. The **medial lemniscus** contains crossed fibers from gracile and cuneate nuclei.

        3. **Pyramid** (corticospinal tracts)

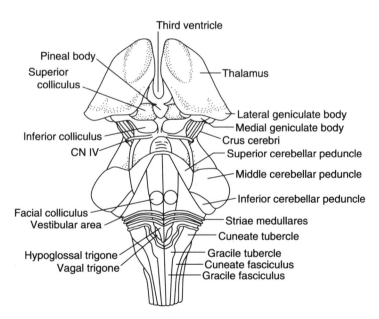

Figure 9-1. Dorsal surface of the brain stem. The three cerebellar peduncles have been removed to expose the rhomboid fossa.

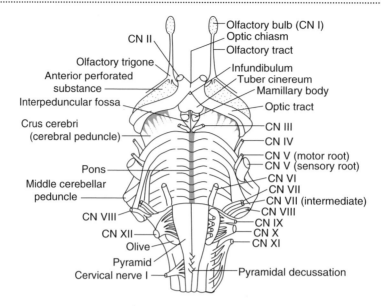

Figure 9-2.   Ventral surface of the brain stem and attached cranial nerves.

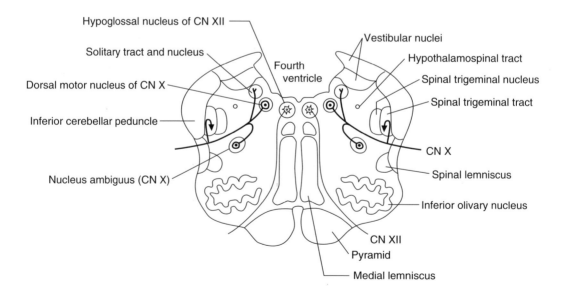

Figure 9-3.   Transverse section of the medulla at the midolivary level. The vagal nerve (CN X), the hypoglossal nerve (CN XII), and the vestibular nerve (CN VIII) are prominent in this section. The nucleus ambiguus gives rise to special visceral efferent fibers to CN IX, CN X, and CN XI.

B. Lateral structures

   1. Nucleus ambiguus (CNN IX, X, and XI)

   2. Vestibular nuclei (CN VIII)

   3. The **inferior cerebellar peduncle** contains the dorsal spinocerebellar, cuneocerebellar, and olivocerebellar tracts.

   4. Lateral spinothalamic tract (spinal lemniscus)

   5. Spinal trigeminal nucleus and tract of CN V

III. CROSS SECTION THROUGH THE PONS (Figure 9-4). The pons has a dorsal tegmentum and a ventral base.

A. Medial structures

   1. Medial longitudinal fasciculus (MLF)

   2. Abducent nucleus of CN VI

   3. Genu (internal) of facial nerve (CN VII)

   4. Abducent fibers of CN VI

   5. Medial lemniscus

   6. Corticospinal tract (in base of pons)

B. Lateral structures

   1. Facial nucleus (CN VII)

   2. Facial (intraaxial) nerve fibers

   3. Spinal trigeminal nucleus and tract (CN V)

   4. Lateral spinothalamic tract (spinal lemniscus)

   5. Vestibular nuclei of CN VIII

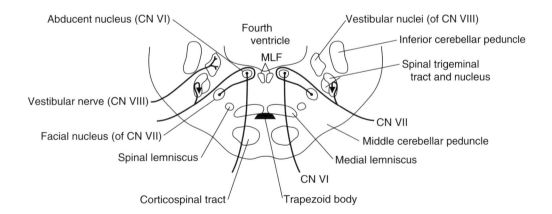

Figure 9-4.   Transverse section of the pons at the level of the abducent nucleus of CN VI and the facial nucleus of CN VII.

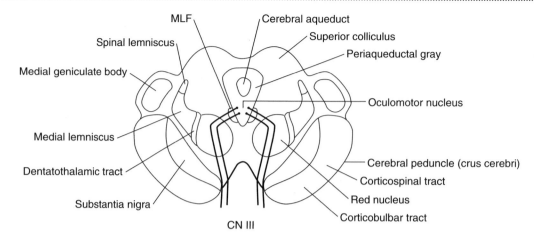

Figure 9-5. Transverse section of the midbrain at the level of the superior colliculus, the oculomotor nucleus (of CN III), and the red nucleus.

IV. CROSS SECTION THROUGH THE ROSTRAL MIDBRAIN (Figure 9-5). The midbrain has a dorsal tectum, an intermediate tegmentum, and a base. The aqueduct lies between the tectum and the tegmentum.

  A. Dorsal structures include the **superior colliculi**.

  B. Tegmentum

    1. Oculomotor nucleus (CN III)

    2. MLF

    3. Red nucleus

    4. Substantia nigra

    5. Dentatothalamic tract (crossed)

    6. Medial lemniscus

    7. Lateral spinothalamic tract (in spinal lemniscus)

  C. Crus cerebri (basis pedunculi or cerebral peduncle). The **corticospinal tract** lies in the middle three-fifths of the crus cerebri.

V. CORTICOBULBAR FIBERS (see also Figure 13-4) project bilaterally to all motor cranial nerve nuclei except the facial nucleus. The division of the facial nerve nucleus that innervates the **upper face** (the orbicularis oculi muscle and above) **receives bilateral corticobulbar input;** the division of the facial nerve nucleus that innervates the **lower face receives** only **contralateral corticobulbar input.**

10

Trigeminal System

I. OVERVIEW.
The trigeminal system provides **sensory innervation to the face, oral cavity, and supratentorial dura** via general somatic afferent (GSA) fibers. It also **innervates the muscles of mastication** via special visceral efferent (SVE) fibers.

II. THE TRIGEMINAL GANGLION
(semilunar or gasserian) contains pseudounipolar ganglion cells. It consists of three divisions:

A. The **ophthalmic nerve (CN V-1)** lies in the wall of the cavernous sinus. It enters the orbit via the superior orbital fissure and innervates the forehead, dorsum of the nose, upper eyelid, orbit (cornea and conjunctiva), and the cranial dura. The ophthalmic nerve mediates the afferent limb of the corneal reflex.

B. The **maxillary nerve (CN V-2)** lies in the wall of the cavernous sinus and innervates the upper lip and cheek, lower eyelid, anterior portion of the temple, oral mucosa of the upper mouth, nose, pharynx, gums, teeth and palate of the upper jaw, and the cranial dura. It exits the skull via the foramen rotundum.

C. The **mandibular nerve (CN V-3)** exits the skull via the foramen ovale.

1. Its **sensory (GSA) component** innervates the lower lip and chin, posterior portion of the temple, external auditory meatus and tympanic membrane, external ear, teeth of the lower jaw, oral mucosa of the cheeks and floor of the mouth, anterior two-thirds of the tongue, temporomandibular joint, and the cranial dura.

2. Its **motor (SVE) component** innervates the muscles of mastication, mylohyoid, anterior belly of the digastric, and the tensores tympani and veli palatini.

III. TRIGEMINOTHALAMIC PATHWAYS (Figure 10-1)

A. The **ventral trigeminothalamic tract** mediates pain and temperature sensation from the face and oral cavity.

1. **First-order neurons** are located in the trigeminal (gasserian) ganglion. They give rise to axons that descend in the spinal trigeminal tract and synapse with second-order neurons in the spinal trigeminal nucleus.

2. **Second-order neurons** are located in the spinal trigeminal nucleus. They give rise to decussating axons that terminate in the contralateral ventral posteromedial (VPM) nucleus of the thalamus.

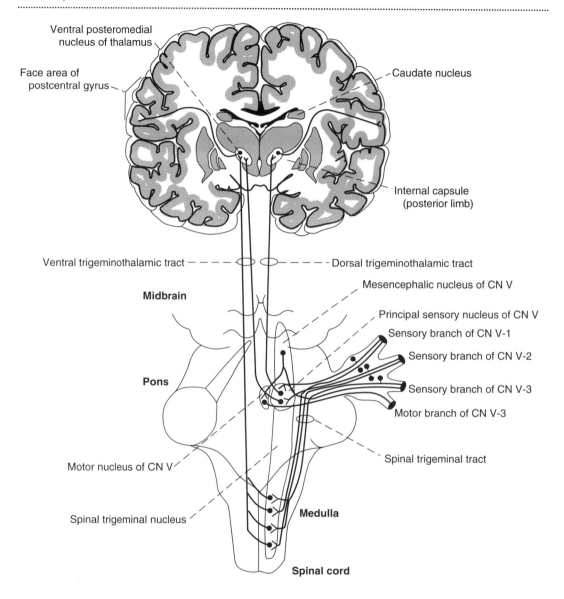

Ventral posteromedial
nucleus of thalamus

Face area of
postcentral gyrus

Caudate nucleus

Internal capsule
(posterior limb)

Ventral trigeminothalamic tract — — — —

Dorsal trigeminothalamic tract

Midbrain

Mesencephalic nucleus of CN V

Principal sensory nucleus of CN V

Sensory branch of CN V-1

Sensory branch of CN V-2

Pons

Sensory branch of CN V-3

Motor branch of CN V-3

Spinal trigeminal tract

Motor nucleus of CN V

Spinal trigeminal nucleus

Medulla

Spinal cord

Figure 10-1. Diagram of the ventral (pain and temperature) and dorsal (discriminative touch) trigemino-thalamic pathways.

>   **3. Third-order neurons** are located in the VPM nucleus of the thalamus. They project via the posterior limb of the internal capsule to the face area of the somatosensory cortex (Brodmann's areas 3, 1, and 2).

> **B.** The **dorsal trigeminothalamic tract** mediates tactile discrimination and pressure sensation from the face and oral cavity. It receives input from Meissner's and Pacini's corpuscles.

>   **1. First-order neurons** are located in the trigeminal (gasserian) ganglion. They synapse in the principal sensory nucleus of CN V.

Table 10-1
Trigeminal Reflexes

Reflex	Afferent Limb	Efferent Limb
Corneal reflex	Ophthalmic nerve (CN V-1)	Facial nerve (CN VII)
Jaw jerk	Mandibular nerve (CN V-3)*	Mandibular nerve (CN V-3)
Tearing (lacrimal) reflex	Ophthalmic nerve (CN V-1)	Facial nerve (CN VII)
Oculocardiac reflex	Ophthalmic nerve (CN V-1)	Vagal nerve (CN X)

*The cell bodies are found in the mesencephalic nucleus of CN V.

2. **Second-order neurons** are located in the principal sensory nucleus of CN V. They project to the ipsilateral VPM nucleus of the thalamus.

3. **Third-order neurons** are located in the VPM nucleus of the thalamus. They project via the posterior limb of the internal capsule to the face area of the somatosensory cortex (Brodmann's areas 3, 1, and 2).

IV. TRIGEMINAL REFLEXES

A. Introduction (Table 10-1)

1. **Corneal reflex** is a consensual and disynaptic reflex.

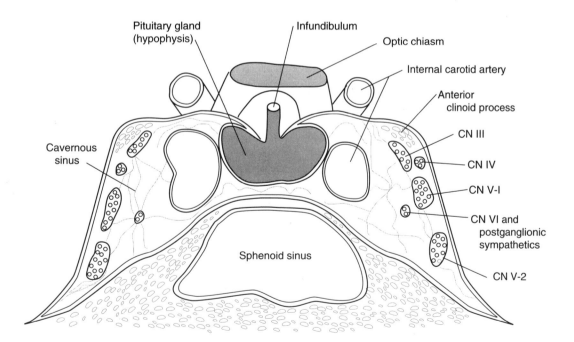

Figure 10-2.   Diagram of the contents of the cavernous sinus. The wall of the cavernous sinus contains the ophthalmic (CN V-1) and maxillary (CN V-2) divisions of the trigeminal nerve (CN V) and the trochlear (CN IV) and oculomotor (CN III) nerves. The siphon of the internal carotid artery and the abducent nerve (CN VI) along with postganglionic sympathetic fibers lie within the cavernous sinus.

   2. **Jaw jerk** is a monosynaptic myotatic reflex.

   3. **Tearing (lacrimal) reflex**

   4. **Oculocardiac reflex.** Pressure on the globe results in **bradycardia**.

B. **Clinical correlation. Trigeminal neuralgia** (tic douloureux) is characterized by recurrent paroxysms of sharp, stabbing pain in one or more branches of the trigeminal nerve on one side of the face. It usually occurs in people older than 50 years, and it is more common in women than in men. **Carbamazepine** is the drug of choice for idiopathic trigeminal neuralgia.

V. THE CAVERNOUS SINUS (Figure 10-2) contains the following structures:

A. **Internal carotid artery** (siphon)

B. **Cranial nerves III, IV, V-1, V-2, and VI**

C. **Postganglionic sympathetic fibers** en route to orbit

11

Auditory System

I. OVERVIEW. The auditory system is an exteroceptive special somatic afferent (SSA) system that can detect sound frequencies from 20 Hz to 20,000 Hz. It is derived from the **otic vesicle,** which is a derivative of the **otic placode,** which is a thickening of the **surface ectoderm**.

II. THE AUDITORY PATHWAY (Figure 11-1) consists of the following structures:

A. Hair cells of the organ of Corti are innervated by the peripheral processes of bipolar cells of the spiral ganglion. They are stimulated by vibrations of the basilar membrane.

B. Bipolar cells of the spiral (cochlear) ganglion project peripherally to hair cells of the organ of Corti. They project centrally as the cochlear nerve to the cochlear nuclei.

C. The **cochlear nerve (CN VIII)** extends from the spiral ganglion to the cerebellopontine angle, where it enters the brain stem.

D. The **cochlear nuclei** receive input from the cochlear nerve. They project contralaterally to the superior olivary nucleus and the lateral lemniscus.

E. The **superior olivary nucleus,** which plays a role in sound localization, receives input from the cochlear nuclei. It projects to the lateral lemniscus.

F. The **trapezoid body** is located in the pons. It contains decussating fibers from the ventral cochlear nuclei.

G. The **lateral lemniscus** receives input from the contralateral cochlear nuclei and from the superior olivary nuclei.

H. The **nucleus of inferior colliculus** receives input from the lateral lemniscus. It projects via the brachium of the inferior colliculus to the medial geniculate body.

I. The **medial geniculate body** receives input from the nucleus of inferior colliculus. It projects via the internal capsule as the auditory radiation to the primary auditory cortex, the transverse gyri of Heschl.

J. The **transverse temporal gyri of Heschl** contain the primary auditory cortex (Brodmann's areas 41 and 42). The gyri are located in the depths of the lateral sulcus.

III. HEARING DEFECTS

A. Conduction deafness is caused by interruption of the passage of sound waves through the external or middle ear. It may be caused by **obstruction** (e.g., wax), **otosclerosis,** or **otitis media**.

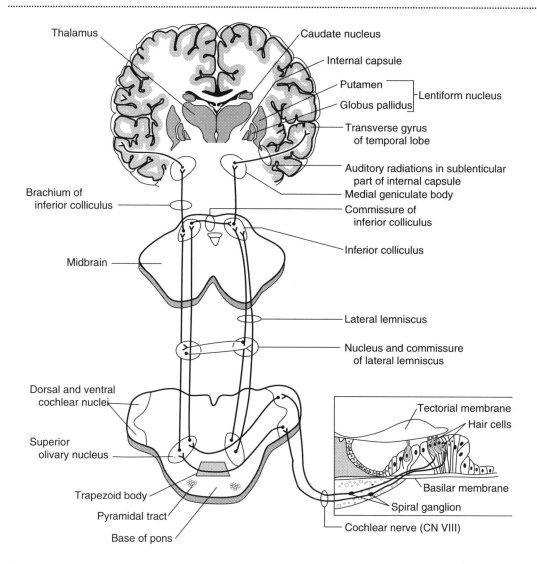

Figure 11-1. Peripheral and central connections of the auditory system. This system arises from the hair cells of the organ of Corti and terminates in the transverse temporal gyri of Heschl of the superior temporal gyrus. It is characterized by bilaterality of projections and tonotopic localization of pitch at all levels (e.g., high pitch, 20,000 Hz, is localized at the base of the cochlea and in the posteromedial part of the transverse temporal gyri).

B. Nerve deafness (sensorineural or perceptive deafness) is caused by disease of the cochlea, cochlear nerve (acoustic neuroma), or central auditory connections. It is most frequently caused by **presbycusis** resulting from degenerative disease of the organ of Corti in the first few millimeters of the basal coil of the cochlea (high-frequency loss of 4,000 Hz to 8,000 Hz).

IV. AUDITORY TESTS

A. Tuning fork tests

1. **Weber's test** is performed by placing a vibrating tuning fork on the vertex of the skull. Normally, a patient hears equally on both sides.

   a. A patient with **unilateral conduction deafness** hears the vibration louder in the diseased ear.

   b. A patient with **unilateral partial nerve deafness** hears the vibration louder in the normal ear.

2. The **Rinne test** compares air and bone conduction. It is performed by placing a vibrating tuning fork on the mastoid process until it is no longer heard; then it is held in front of the ear. Normally, a patient hears vibration in the air after bone conduction is gone.

   a. A patient with **unilateral conduction deafness** fails to hear vibrations in the air after bone conduction is gone.

   b. A patient with **unilateral partial nerve deafness** hears vibrations in the air after bone conduction is gone.

B. Brain stem auditory evoked potentials (BAEPs)

1. **Test method.** Clicks are presented to one ear, then to the other. Scalp electrodes and a computer generate a series of seven waves that can be associated with areas of the auditory pathway.

2. **Diagnostic value.** This method is valuable for diagnosing brain stem lesions (**multiple sclerosis**), diagnosing posterior fossa tumors (**acoustic neuromas**), and assessing hearing in infants. Approximately 50% of patients with multiple sclerosis show abnormalities of the BAEPs.

12

Vestibular System

I. OVERVIEW. Like the auditory system, the vestibular system is derived from the **otic vesicle,** which is a derivative of the **otic placode,** which is a thickening of the **surface ectoderm.** This system maintains **posture** and **equilibrium** and coordinates **head and eye movements.**

II. LABYRINTH

    A. Kinetic labyrinth

        1. Three semicircular ducts lie within the three semicircular canals (i.e., the superior, lateral, and posterior canals).

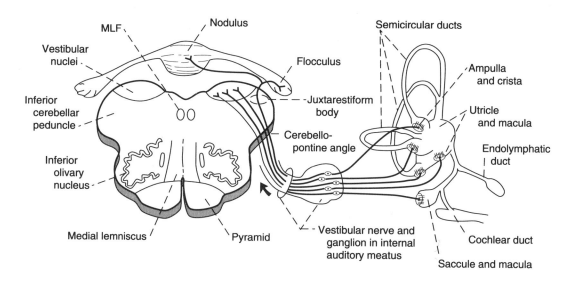

Figure 12-1. Peripheral connections of the vestibular system. Hair cells of the cristae ampullares and the maculae of the utricle and saccule project, via the vestibular nerve, to the vestibular nuclei of the medulla and pons and to the flocculonodular lobe of the cerebellum (vestibulocerebellum).

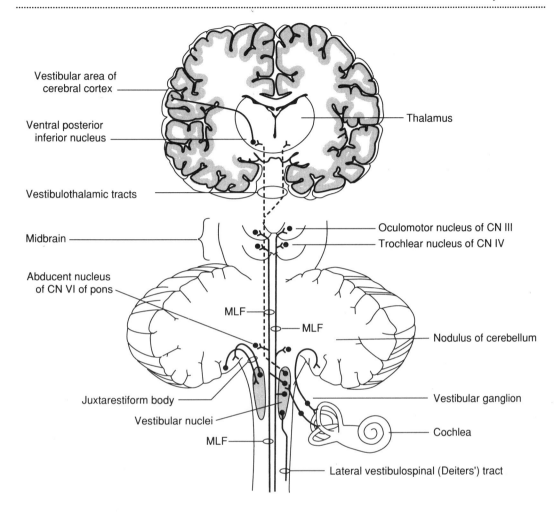

Vestibular area of cerebral cortex

Ventral posterior inferior nucleus

Vestibulothalamic tracts

Midbrain

Abducent nucleus of CN VI of pons

MLF

MLF

Juxtarestiform body

Vestibular nuclei

MLF

Thalamus

Oculomotor nucleus of CN III
Trochlear nucleus of CN IV

Nodulus of cerebellum

Vestibular ganglion

Cochlea

Lateral vestibulospinal (Deiters') tract

Figure 12-2. Major central connections of the vestibular system. Vestibular nuclei project via the ascending medial longitudinal fasciculi (MLF) to the ocular motor nuclei and subserve vestibulo-ocular reflexes. Vestibular nuclei project, via the descending MLF and the lateral vestibulospinal tracts, to the ventral horn motor neurons of the spinal cord and mediate postural reflexes.

2. These ducts **respond to angular acceleration and deceleration of the head**.
   a. They contain **hair cells** in the crista ampullaris that **respond to endolymph flow**.
   b. Endolymph flow toward the ampulla (ampullopetal) or utricle (utriculopetal) is a stronger stimulus than is endolymph flow in the opposite direction.

B. Static labyrinth

1. The **utricle and saccule** respond to the position of the head with respect to **linear acceleration** and the pull of **gravity**.

2. The utricle and saccule contain **hair cells** whose cilia are embedded in the otolithic membrane. When hair cells are bent toward the longest cilium (kinocilium), the frequency of sensory discharge increases.

III. **VESTIBULAR PATHWAYS** (Figures 12-1 and 12-2) consist of the following structures:

A. **Hair cells of the semicircular ducts and of the saccule and utricle** are innervated by peripheral processes of **bipolar cells** of the vestibular ganglion.

B. The **vestibular ganglion** is located in the fundus of the internal auditory meatus.

1. Bipolar neurons project via their peripheral processes to the hair cells.

2. Bipolar neurons project their central processes, as the vestibular nerve (CN VIII) to the vestibular nuclei, and to the flocculonodular lobe of the cerebellum.

C. Vestibular nuclei

1. Receive input from:
   a. Semicircular ducts, the saccule, and the utricle
   b. Flocculonodular lobe of the cerebellum

2. Project fibers to:
   a. Flocculonodular lobe of cerebellum
   b. CN III, CN IV, and CN VI via the medial longitudinal fasciculus (MLF)
   c. Spinal cord via the lateral vestibulospinal tract
   d. Ventral posteroinferior (VPI) and ventral posterolateral (VPL) nuclei of the thalamus, both of which project to the postcentral gyrus

IV. **VESTIBULO-OCULAR REFLEXES** are mediated by the vestibular nuclei, the MLF, ocular motor nuclei, and CNs III, IV, and VI.

A. Vestibular nystagmus (horizontal nystagmus)

1. **Fast phase** of nystagmus is in the **direction of rotation.**

2. **Slow phase** of nystagmus is in the **opposite direction.**

B. Postrotatory nystagmus (horizontal nystagmus)

1. **Fast phase** of nystagmus is **opposite the direction of rotation.**

2. **Slow phase** of nystagmus is in the **direction of rotation.**

3. The patient will past point and fall in the direction of prior rotation.

C. Caloric nystagmus (stimulation of horizontal ducts)

1. **Cold water irrigation** of the external auditory meatus results in nystagmus to the opposite side.

2. **Warm water irrigation** of the external auditory meatus results in nystagmus to the same side.

3. Remember the mnemonic **"COWS":** cold opposite, warm same.

13

Cranial Nerves

I. OLFACTORY NERVE. The olfactory nerve, the first cranial nerve (**CN I;** Figure 13-1), mediates olfaction (**smell**). It is the only sensory system that has no precortical relay in the thalamus. The olfactory nerve, which is a special visceral afferent (SVA) nerve, consists of unmyelinated axons of bipolar neurons located in the nasal mucosa, the olfactory epithelium. It enters the skull via the cribriform plate of the ethmoid bone. (See appendix for a table of cranial nerves.)

A. Olfactory pathway

1. Olfactory receptor cells are first-order neurons that project to the mitral cells of the olfactory bulb.

2. Mitral cells are the principal cells of the olfactory bulb. They are excitatory and glutaminergic. They project via the **olfactory tract** and **lateral olfactory stria** to the primary olfactory cortex and to the amygdala.

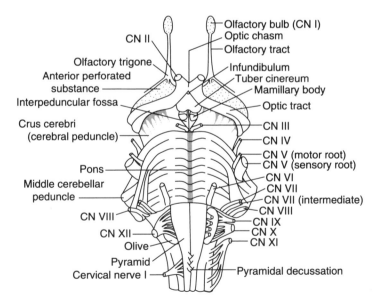

Figure 13-1. Base of the brain with attached cranial nerves. (Reprinted with permission from Truex RC and Kellner CE: *Detailed Atlas of the Head and Neck.* New York, Oxford University Press, 1958, p 34.)

3. Primary olfactory cortex (area 34) consists of the piriform cortex that overlies the uncus.

B. Lesions of the olfactory pathway result from trauma (e.g., skull fracture) and, frequently, from olfactory groove meningiomas. These lesions **result in ipsilateral anosmia** (localizing value). Lesions involving the parahippocampal uncus may cause olfactory hallucinations [uncinate fits (seizures) with déjà vu].

II. OPTIC NERVE. The optic nerve, CN II (SSA), subserves vision and pupillary light reflexes (afferent limb) [see Chapter 19]. It is **not** a true **peripheral nerve** but is a tract of the diencephalon; a transected optic nerve cannot regenerate.

III. OCULOMOTOR NERVE. The oculomotor nerve (**CN III**) is a GSE, GVE nerve.

A. General characteristics of CN III. The oculomotor nerve **moves the eye, constricts the pupil, accommodates, and converges.** It exits the brain stem from the interpeduncular fossa of the midbrain, passes through the cavernous sinus, and enters the orbit via the superior orbital fissure.

1. The **GSE component** arises from the oculomotor nucleus of the rostral midbrain. It innervates four extraocular muscles and the levator palpebrae muscle. (Remember the mnemonic **SIN**: Superior muscles are **IN**torters of the globe.)
   a. The **medial rectus muscle** adducts the eye. With its opposite partner, it converges the eyes.
   b. The **superior rectus muscle** elevates, intorts, and adducts the eye.
   c. The **inferior rectus muscle** depresses, extorts, and adducts the eye.
   d. The **inferior oblique muscle** elevates, extorts, and abducts the eye.
   e. The **levator palpebrae muscle** elevates the upper lid.

2. The **GVE component** consists of preganglionic parasympathetic fibers.
   a. The **Edinger-Westphal nucleus** projects preganglionic parasympathetic fibers to the ciliary ganglion of the orbit via CN III.
   b. The **ciliary ganglion** projects postganglionic parasympathetic fibers to the sphincter muscle of the iris (miosis) and to the ciliary muscle (accommodation).

B. Clinical correlations of CN III

1. Oculomotor paralysis (palsy) is seen with transtentorial herniation (e.g., tumor, subdural or epidural hematoma).
   a. Denervation of the levator palpebrae muscle results in **ptosis** (drooping of the upper eyelid).
   b. Denervation of the extraocular muscles causes the affected eye to "look down and out" due to the unopposed action of the lateral rectus and superior oblique muscles. The superior oblique and lateral rectus muscles are innervated by CN IV and CN VI, respectively. Oculomotor palsy results in **diplopia** (double vision) when the patient looks in the direction of the paretic muscle.
   c. Interruption of parasympathetic innervation (internal ophthalmoplegia) results in a **dilated and fixed pupil and paralysis of accommodation** (cycloplegia).

2. Other conditions associated with CN III impairment
   a. Transtentorial (uncal) herniation. Increased supratentorial pressure (e.g., from a tumor) forces the hippocampal uncus through the tentorial notch and compresses or stretches the oculomotor nerve.

(1) **Pupilloconstrictor fibers** are affected first, resulting in a **dilated and fixed pupil**.

(2) **Somatic efferent fibers** are affected later, resulting in an **external strabismus** (exotropia).

b. Aneurysms of the carotid and posterior communicating arteries frequently compress CN III within the cavernous sinus or the interpeduncular cistern. They usually affect the peripheral pupilloconstrictor fibers first, as in uncal herniation.

c. Diabetes mellitus (diabetic oculomotor palsy) frequently affects the oculomotor nerve, damaging the central fibers and sparing the pupilloconstrictor fibers.

IV. TROCHLEAR NERVE. The trochlear nerve (CN IV) is a GSE nerve.

A. General characteristics. The trochlear nerve is a pure motor nerve that innervates the superior oblique muscle, which depresses, intorts, and abducts the eye.

1. It **arises from** the contralateral trochlear nucleus of the caudal midbrain.

2. It **decussates** beneath the superior medullary velum of the midbrain and exits the brain stem on its dorsal surface, caudal to the inferior colliculus.

3. It **encircles the midbrain** within the subarachnoid space, passes through the cavernous sinus, and enters the orbit via the superior orbital fissure.

B. Clinical correlation. CN IV paralysis results in the following conditions:

1. Extorsion of the eye and weakness of downward gaze

2. Vertical diplopia, which increases when looking down

3. Head tilting, which is done to compensate for extorsion (this may be misdiagnosed as idiopathic torticollis)

4. Head trauma. The trochlear nerve, due to its course around the midbrain, is particularly vulnerable to head trauma.

V. TRIGEMINAL NERVE. The trigeminal nerve (CN V) is an SVE, GSA nerve (see Chapter 10).

A. General characteristics of CN V. The trigeminal nerve is the nerve of pharyngeal (branchial) arch 1 (mandibular). It has three divisions: ophthalmic (CN V-1), maxillary (CN V-2), and mandibular (CN V-3) [see Chapter 10].

1. The **SVE component** arises from the motor trigeminal nucleus found in the lateral midpontine tegmentum. It **innervates the muscles of mastication** (i.e., the temporalis, masseter, lateral, and medial pterygoids), the tensores tympani and veli palatini, the myelohyoid muscle, and the anterior belly of the digastric muscle.

2. The **GSA component** provides **sensory innervation to the face,** mucous membranes of the nasal and oral cavities and frontal sinus, hard palate, and deep structures of the head (proprioception from muscles and the temporomandibular joint). It innervates the dura of the anterior and middle cranial fossae (supratentorial dura).

B. Clinical correlation. Lesions of CN V result in the following neurological deficits:

1. Loss of general sensation (**hemianesthesia**) from the face and mucous membranes of the oral and nasal cavities

2. Loss of the corneal reflex (afferent limb, CN V-1) [Figure 13-2]

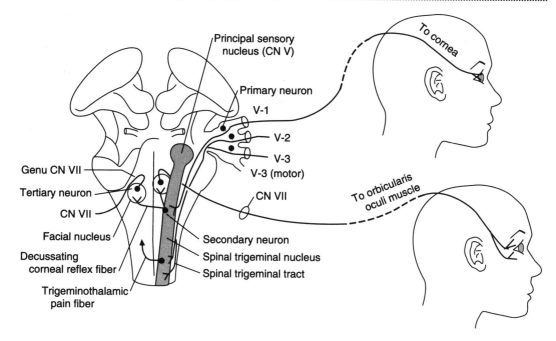

Figure 13-2. Corneal reflex pathway showing the three neurons and decussation. This reflex is consensual like the pupillary light reflex. Note that second-order pain neurons are found in the caudal division of the spinal trigeminal nucleus. Second-order corneal reflex neurons are found at more rostral levels.

3. **Flaccid paralysis** of the muscles of mastication

4. **Deviation of the patient's jaw to the weak side,** because of the unopposed action of the opposite lateral pterygoid muscle

5. **Paralysis of the tensor tympani muscle,** leading to hypoacusis (partial deafness to low-pitched sounds)

6. **Trigeminal neuralgia** (tic douloureux), which is characterized by recurrent paroxysms of sharp, stabbing pain in one or more branches of the nerve (see Chapter 10)

VI. ABDUCENT NERVE (CN VI)

A. **General characteristics.** The abducent nerve is a pure **GSE nerve** that innervates the lateral rectus muscle, which abducts the eye.

1. It arises from the abducent nucleus found in the dorsomedial tegmentum of the caudal pons.

2. Exiting intra-axial fibers pass through the corticospinal tract. **A lesion results in an alternating abducent hemiparesis.**

3. It passes through the pontine cistern and the cavernous sinus and enters the orbit via the superior orbital fissure.

B. **Clinical correlation. CN VI paralysis** is the most common isolated palsy resulting from the long peripheral course of the nerve. It is seen in patients with meningitis, subarachnoid hemorrhage, late syphilis, and trauma. Abducent nerve paralysis **results in the following defects**:

1. **Convergent (medial) strabismus (esotropia)** with the inability to abduct the eye

2. **Horizontal diplopia** with maximum separation of the double images when looking toward the paretic lateral rectus muscle

VII. FACIAL NERVE (CN VII)

A. General characteristics. The facial nerve is a **GSA, GVA, SVA, GVE,** and **SVE** nerve (Figures 13-3 and 13-4). It **mediates facial movements, taste, salivation, lacrimation, and general sensation from the external ear**. It is the nerve of pharyngeal (branchial) arch 2 (hyoid). It includes the facial nerve proper (motor division), which contains the SVE fibers that **innervate the muscles of facial (mimetic) expression.** CN VII includes the intermediate nerve, which contains GSA, SVA, and GVE fibers. All first-order sensory neurons are found in the geniculate ganglion within the temporal bone.

1. **Anatomy.** The facial nerve exits the brain stem in the cerebellopontine angle. It enters the internal auditory meatus and the facial canal. It then exits the facial canal and skull via the stylomastoid foramen.

2. The **GSA component** has cell bodies located in the geniculate ganglion. It innervates the posterior surface of the external ear via the posterior auricular branch of CN VII. It projects centrally to the spinal trigeminal tract and nucleus.

3. The **GVA component** is clinically worthless. Cell bodies are located in the geniculate ganglion. Fibers innervate the soft palate and adjacent pharyngeal wall.

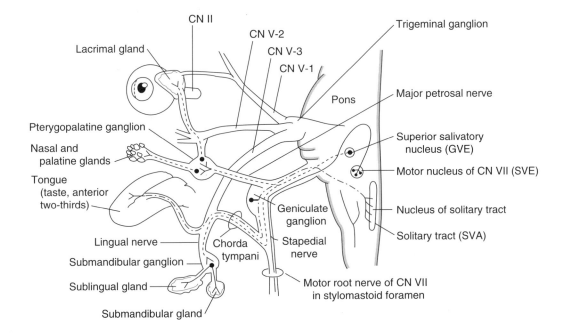

Figure 13-3. The functional components of the facial nerve (CN VII).

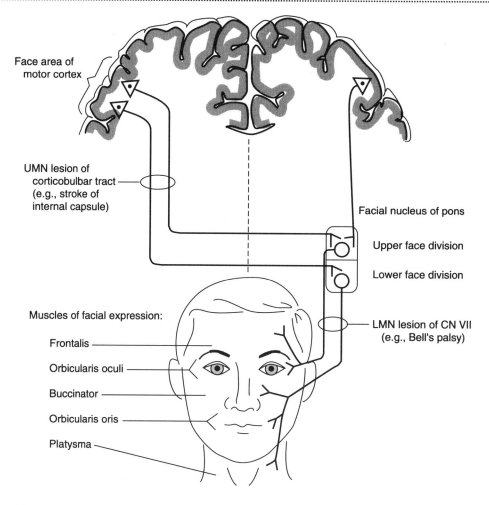

Figure 13-4. Corticobulbar innervation of the facial nerve (CN VII) nucleus. An upper motor neuron (UMN) lesion (e.g., a stroke involving the internal capsule) results in contralateral weakness of the lower face and spares the upper face. A lower motor neuron (LMN) lesion (e.g., Bell's palsy) results in paralysis of facial muscles in both the upper and the lower face.

4. The **SVA component (taste)** has cell bodies located in the geniculate ganglion. It projects centrally to the solitary tract and nucleus. It innervates the taste buds from the anterior two-thirds of the tongue via:
    a. Intermediate nerve
    b. Chorda tympani, which is located in the tympanic cavity medial to the tympanic membrane and malleus. It contains the SVA and GVE (parasympathetic) fibers.
    c. Lingual nerve (a branch of CN V-3)
    d. Central gustatory pathway (see Figure 13-3). Taste fibers from CN VII, CN IX, and CN X project via the solitary tract to the solitary nucleus. The solitary nucleus projects via the central tegmental tract to the ventral posteromedial nucleus (VPM) of the thalamus. The VPM projects to the gustatory cortex of the parietal lobe (parietal operculum).

5. The **GVE component** is a parasympathetic component that innervates the lacrimal, submandibular, and sublingual glands. It contains preganglionic parasympathetic neurons located in the superior salivatory nucleus of the caudal pons.

    a. Lacrimal pathway (see Figure 13-3). The superior salivatory nucleus projects via the intermediate and greater petrosal nerves to the pterygopalatine (sphenopalatine) ganglion. The pterygopalatine ganglion projects to the lacrimal gland of the orbit.

    b. Submandibular pathway (see Figure 13-3). The superior salivatory nucleus projects via the intermediate nerve and chorda tympani to the submandibular ganglion. The submandibular ganglion projects to and innervates the submandibular and sublingual glands.

6. The **SVE component** arises from the facial nucleus, loops around the abducent nucleus of the caudal pons, and exits the brain stem in the cerebellopontine angle. It enters the internal auditory meatus, traverses the facial canal, sends a branch to the stapedius muscle of the middle ear, and exits the skull via the stylomastoid foramen. It innervates the muscles of facial expression, the stylohyoid muscle, the posterior belly of the digastric muscle, and the stapedius muscle.

B. Clinical correlation. Lesions of CN VII (see Figure 14-2) result in the following conditions:

1. Flaccid **paralysis of the muscles of facial expression** (upper and lower face)

2. Loss of the corneal reflex (efferent limb), which may lead to corneal ulceration

3. Loss of taste from the anterior two-thirds of the tongue, which may result from damage to the chorda tympani

4. Hyperacusis (increased acuity to sounds), due to stapedius paralysis

5. Bell's palsy (peripheral facial paralysis), which is caused by trauma or infection and involves the upper and lower face

6. Crocodile tears syndrome (lacrimation during eating), which is a result of aberrant regeneration after trauma

7. Supranuclear (central) facial palsy, which is associated with ipsilateral hemiplegia and spares the corrugator, frontalis, and orbicularis oculi muscles

8. Bilateral facial nerve palsies, which occur in Guillain-Barré syndrome (see Chapter 14)

VIII. VESTIBULOCOCHLEAR NERVE (CN VIII). The vestibulocochlear nerve is an SSA nerve.

It consists of two functional divisions: the vestibular nerve, which **maintains equilibrium and balance,** and the cochlear nerve, which **mediates hearing** (see Chapters 11 and 12). It exits the brain stem at the cerebellopontine angle. It enters the internal auditory meatus and is confined to the temporal bone.

A. Vestibular nerve (see Figure 12-1)

1. General characteristics. The vestibular nerve:

    a. is associated functionally with the cerebellum (flocculonodular lobe) and ocular motor nuclei

    b. regulates compensatory eye movements

    c. has its first-order sensory bipolar neurons in the vestibular ganglion in the fundus of the internal auditory meatus

  d. projects its peripheral processes to the hair cells of the cristae of the semicircular ducts and to hair cells of the utricle and saccule

  e. projects its central processes to the four vestibular nuclei of the brain stem and to the flocculonodular lobe of the cerebellum

  f. conducts efferent fibers to the hair cells from the brain stem

 2. Clinical correlation. Lesions of the vestibular nerve result in **disequilibrium, vertigo, and nystagmus.**

B. Cochlear nerve (see Figure 11-1)

 1. General characteristics. The cochlear nerve:

  a. has its first-order sensory bipolar neurons in the spiral (cochlear) ganglion of the modiolus of the cochlea, within the temporal bone

  b. projects its peripheral processes to the hair cells of the organ of Corti

  c. projects its central processes to the dorsal and ventral cochlear nuclei of the brain stem

  d. conducts efferent fibers to the hair cells from the brain stem

 2. Clinical correlation. Destructive lesions of the cochlear nerve result in **hearing loss** (sensorineural deafness). Irritative lesions can cause **tinnitus** (ear ringing). An **acoustic neuroma** (schwannoma) is a Schwann cell tumor of the cochlear nerve that causes deafness (see Chapter 14).

IX. GLOSSOPHARYNGEAL NERVE (CN IX). The glossopharyngeal nerve is a **GSA, GVA, SVA, SVE,** and **GVE** nerve.

A. General characteristics. The glossopharyngeal nerve is primarily a sensory nerve. It **mediates taste, salivation, and swallowing** (along with CN X, CN XI, and CN XII). It **mediates input from the carotid sinus,** which contains baroreceptors that monitor arterial blood pressure. It also **mediates input from the carotid body,** which contains chemoreceptors that monitor the CO_2 and O_2 concentration of the blood.

 1. Anatomy. It is the nerve of pharyngeal (branchial) arch 3. It exits the brain stem (medulla) from the postolivary sulcus with CN X and CN XI. It exits the skull via the jugular foramen with CN X and CN XI.

 2. The **GSA component** innervates part of the external ear and the external auditory meatus via the auricular branch of the vagus nerve. It has cell bodies in the superior ganglion. It projects its central processes to the spinal trigeminal tract and nucleus.

 3. The **GVA component** innervates structures derived from the endoderm (e.g., the pharynx). It **innervates the mucous membranes** of the posterior one-third of the tongue, tonsil, upper pharynx, tympanic cavity, and auditory tube. It also **innervates the carotid sinus** (baroreceptors) **and the carotid body** (chemoreceptors) via the sinus nerve. It has cell bodies in the inferior (petrosal) ganglion. It is the afferent limb of the gag reflex and the carotid sinus reflex.

 4. The **SVA component** innervates the taste buds of the posterior one-third of the tongue. It has cell bodies in the inferior (petrosal) ganglion. It projects its central processes to the solitary tract and nucleus (for central pathway, see VII).

 5. The **SVE component** innervates only the stylopharyngeus muscle. It arises from the nucleus ambiguus of the lateral medulla.

 6. The **GVE component** is a parasympathetic component that innervates the parotid gland. Preganglionic parasympathetic neurons are located in the inferior salivatory nucleus of the medulla; they project via the tympanic and lesser petrosal nerves to the otic ganglion. Postganglionic fibers from the otic ganglion project to the parotid gland via the auriculotemporal nerve (CN V-3).

B. **Clinical correlation. Lesions of CN IX** result in the following conditions:

1. **Loss of the gag (pharyngeal) reflex** (interruption of the afferent limb)

2. **Hypersensitive carotid sinus reflex** (syncope)

3. **Loss of general sensation in the pharynx, tonsils, fauces, and back of the tongue**

4. **Loss of taste** from the posterior one-third of the tongue

5. **Glossopharyngeal neuralgia** is characterized by severe stabbing pain in the root of the tongue.

X. VAGAL NERVE (CN X). The vagal nerve is a **GSA, GVA, SVA, SVE, and GVE** nerve.

A. **General characteristics.** The vagal nerve **mediates phonation, swallowing** (with CN IX, CN XI, CN XII), elevation of the palate, taste, and cutaneous sensation from the ear. It **innervates the viscera of the neck, thorax, and abdomen.**

1. **Anatomy.** The vagal nerve is the nerve of pharyngeal (branchial) arches 4 and 6 (pharyngeal arch 5 is either absent or rudimentary). It exits the brain stem (medulla) from the postolivary sulcus. It exits the skull via the jugular foramen with CN IX and CN XI.

2. The **GSA component** innervates the infratentorial dura, external ear, external auditory meatus, and tympanic membrane. It has cell bodies in the superior (jugular) ganglion. It projects its central processes to the spinal trigeminal tract and nucleus.

3. The **GVA component** innervates the mucous membranes of the pharynx, larynx, esophagus, trachea, and thoracic and abdominal viscera (to the left colic flexure). It has cell bodies in the inferior (nodose) ganglion. It projects its central processes to the solitary tract and nucleus.

4. The **SVA component** innervates the taste buds in the epiglottic region. It has cell bodies in the inferior (nodose) ganglion. It projects its central processes to the solitary tract and nucleus. For central pathway, see CN VII.

5. The **SVE component** innervates the pharyngeal (branchial) arch muscles of the larynx and pharynx, striated muscle of the upper esophagus, muscle of the uvula, and the levator veli palatini and palatoglossus muscles. It receives SVE input from the cranial division of the spinal accessory nerve (CN XI). It arises from the nucleus ambiguus in the lateral medulla. The SVE component provides the efferent limb of the gag reflex.

6. The **GVE component** innervates the viscera of the neck and the thoracic (heart) and abdominal cavities as far as the left colic flexure. Preganglionic parasympathetic neurons located in the dorsal motor nucleus of the medulla project to the terminal (intramural) ganglia of the visceral organs.

B. **Clinical correlation. Lesions and reflexes of CN X** result in the following conditions:

1. **Ipsilateral paralysis** of the soft palate, pharynx, and larynx, which leads to dysphonia (hoarseness), dyspnea, dysarthria, and dysphagia

2. **Loss of the gag (palatal) reflex** (efferent limb)

3. **Anesthesia of the pharynx and larynx,** which leads to unilateral loss of the cough reflex

4. **Aortic aneurysms and tumors** of the neck and thorax, which frequently compress the vagal nerve

5. **Complete laryngeal paralysis,** which can be rapidly fatal if paralysis is bilateral (asphyxia)

6. **Parasympathetic (vegetative) disturbances,** which include bradycardia (irritative lesion), tachycardia (destructive lesion), and dilation of the stomach

7. **Oculocardiac reflex,** in which pressure on the eye slows the heart rate (afferent limb of CN V-1; efferent limb of CN X)

8. **Carotid sinus reflex,** in which pressure on the carotid sinus results in slowing of the heart rate (bradycardia; efferent limb of CN X)

XI. ACCESSORY NERVE (spinal accessory nerve; CN XI). The accessory nerve is an SVE nerve.

  A. **General characteristics.** The accessory nerve **mediates head and shoulder movement** and **innervates laryngeal muscles.** It includes the following divisions:

   1. **Cranial division (accessory portion).** The cranial division of the accessory nerve arises from the nucleus ambiguus of the medulla. It exits the medulla from the post-olivary sulcus and joins the vagal nerve, CN X. It exits the skull via the jugular foramen with CN IX and CN X. It **innervates the intrinsic muscles of the larynx** via the inferior (recurrent) laryngeal nerve, with the exception of the cricothyroid muscle.

   2. **Spinal division** (spinal portion). This division of the accessory nerve arises from the ventral horn of cervical segments C1 to C6. Spinal roots exit the spinal cord laterally between the ventral and dorsal spinal roots, ascend through the foramen magnum, and exit the skull via the jugular. It **innervates the sternocleidomastoid muscle** with the cervical plexus (C-2) **and the trapezius muscle** with the cervical plexus (C-3 and C-4).

  B. **Clinical correlation.** Lesions of CN XI result in the following conditions:

   1. **Paralysis of the sternocleidomastoid muscle,** which results in difficulty in turning the head to the contralateral side

   2. **Paralysis of the trapezius muscle,** which results in a shoulder droop and the inability to shrug the shoulder.

   3. **Paralysis of the larynx,** if the cranial root is involved

XII. HYPOGLOSSAL NERVE (CN XII). The hypoglossal nerve is a GSE nerve.

  A. **General characteristics.** The hypoglossal nerve **mediates tongue movement.** It arises from the hypoglossal nucleus of the medulla. It exits the medulla in the preolivary sulcus. It exits the skull via the hypoglossal canal. It **innervates the intrinsic and extrinsic muscles of the tongue.**

  B. **Clinical correlations**

   1. **Transection** results in hemiparalysis of the tongue.

   2. **Protrusion** causes the tongue to point toward the weak side because of the unopposed action of the opposite genioglossus muscle.

14

Lesions of the Brain Stem

I. LESIONS OF THE MEDULLA (Figure 14-1)

A. Medial medullary syndrome (anterior spinal artery syndrome). Affected structures and resultant deficits include:

1. Corticospinal tract (medullary pyramid). Lesions here result in contralateral spastic hemiparesis.

2. Medial lemniscus. Lesions here result in contralateral loss of tactile and vibration sensation from the trunk and extremities.

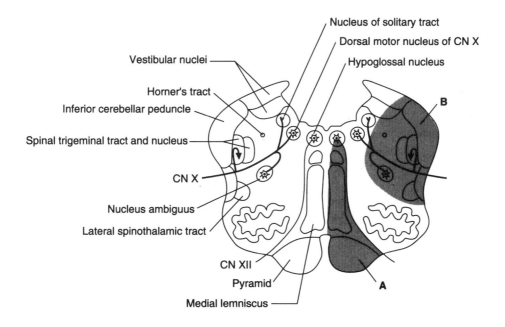

Figure 14-1. Vascular lesions of the caudal medulla at the level of the hypoglossal nucleus of CN XII and the dorsal motor nucleus of CN X. *(A)* Medial medullary syndrome (anterior spinal artery). *(B)* Lateral medullary syndrome (PICA syndrome).

3. **Hypoglossal nucleus or intra-axial root fibers CN XII).** Lesions here result in ipsilateral flaccid hemiparalysis of the tongue. When protruded, the tongue points to the side of the lesion (i.e., to the weak side).

B. **Lateral medullary syndrome [posterior inferior cerebellar artery (PICA) syndrome]** is characterized by dissociated sensory loss (see I B 6–7). Affected structures and resultant deficits include:

1. **Vestibular nuclei.** Lesions here result in nystagmus, nausea, vomiting, and vertigo.

2. **Inferior cerebellar peduncle.** Lesions here result in ipsilateral cerebellar signs [e.g., dystaxia, dysmetria (past pointing), dysdiadochokinesia].

3. **Nucleus ambiguus of CN IX, CN X, and CN XI.** Lesions here result in ipsilateral laryngeal, pharyngeal, and palatal hemiparalysis [i.e., loss of gag reflex (efferent limb), dysarthria, dysphagia, and dysphonia (hoarseness)].

4. **Glossopharyngeal nerve roots.** Lesions here result in loss of the gag reflex (afferent limb).

5. **Vagal nerve roots** (see I B 3)

6. **Spinothalamic tracts (spinal lemniscus).** Lesions of these tracts result in contralateral loss of pain and temperature sensation from the trunk and extremities.

7. **Spinal trigeminal nucleus and tract.** A lesion here results in ipsilateral loss of pain and temperature sensation from the face (facial hemianesthesia).

8. **Descending sympathetic tract.** Lesions here result in ipsilateral Horner's syndrome (ptosis, miosis, hemianhidrosis, and apparent enophthalmos).

II. LESIONS OF THE PONS (Figure 14-2)

A. **Medial inferior pontine syndrome** results from occlusion of the paramedian branches of the basilar artery. Affected structures and resultant deficits include:

1. **Corticospinal tract.** Lesions here result in contralateral spastic hemiparesis.

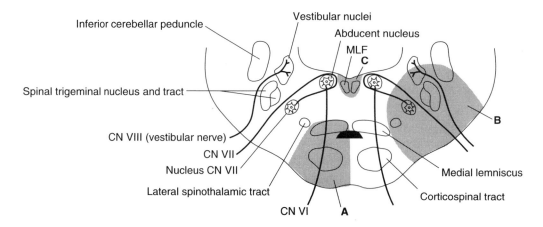

Figure 14-2. Vascular lesions of the caudal pons at the level of the abducent nucleus of CN VI and the facial nucleus of CN VII. (A) Medial inferior pontine syndrome. (B) Lateral inferior pontine syndrome (AICA syndrome). (C) Medial longitudinal fasciculus (MLF) syndrome.

2. Medial lemniscus. Lesions here result in contralateral loss of tactile sensation from the trunk and extremities.

3. Abducent nerve roots. Lesions here result in ipsilateral lateral rectus paralysis.

B. Lateral inferior pontine syndrome [anterior inferior cerebellar artery (AICA) syndrome]. Affected structures and resultant deficits include:

1. **Facial nucleus and intra-axial nerve fibers.** Lesions here result in:
    a. Ipsilateral facial nerve paralysis
    b. Ipsilateral loss of taste from the anterior two-thirds of the tongue
    c. Ipsilateral loss of lacrimation and reduced salivation
    d. Loss of corneal and stapedial reflexes (efferent limbs)

2. **Cochlear nuclei and intra-axial nerve fibers.** Lesions here result in unilateral central deafness.

3. **Vestibular nuclei and intra-axial nerve fibers.** Lesions here result in nystagmus, nausea, vomiting, and vertigo.

4. **Spinal trigeminal nucleus and tract.** Lesions here result in ipsilateral loss of pain and temperature sensation from the face (facial hemianesthesia).

5. **Middle and inferior cerebellar peduncles.** Lesions here result in ipsilateral limb and gait dystaxia.

6. **Spinothalamic tracts (spinal lemniscus).** Lesions here result in contralateral loss of pain and temperature sensation from the trunk and extremities.

7. **Descending sympathetic tract.** Lesions here result in ipsilateral Horner's syndrome.

C. Medial longitudinal fasciculus (MLF) syndrome (internuclear ophthalmoplegia; see Figure 14-2C) interrupts fibers from the contralateral abducent nucleus that project, via the MLF, to the ipsilateral medial rectus subnucleus of CN III. It results in a **medial rectus palsy** on attempted lateral conjugate gaze and **nystagmus** in the abducting eye; convergence remains intact. This syndrome is frequently seen in patients with **multiple sclerosis**.

III. LESIONS OF THE MIDBRAIN (Figure 14-3)

A. Dorsal midbrain (Parinaud) syndrome (see Figure 14-3A) is frequently the result of a pinealoma or germinoma of the pineal region. Affected structures and resultant deficits include:

1. **Superior colliculus and pretectal area.** Lesions here result in paralysis of upward and downward gaze, pupillary disturbances, and absence of convergence.

2. **Cerebral aqueduct.** Compression results in a noncommunicating hydrocephalus.

B. Paramedian midbrain (Benedikt) syndrome (see Figure 14-3B). Affected structures and resultant deficits include:

1. **Oculomotor nerve roots** (intra-axial fibers). Lesions here result in complete ipsilateral oculomotor paralysis; eye abduction and depression are caused by the intact lateral rectus (CN VI) and superior oblique (CN IV). Ptosis (paralysis of the levator palpebrae muscle) and an ipsilateral fixed and dilated pupil (complete internal ophthalmoplegia) also occur.

2. **Dentatothalamic fibers.** Lesions here result in contralateral cerebellar dystaxia with intention tremor.

3. **Medial lemniscus.** Lesions here result in contralateral loss of tactile sensation from the trunk and extremities.

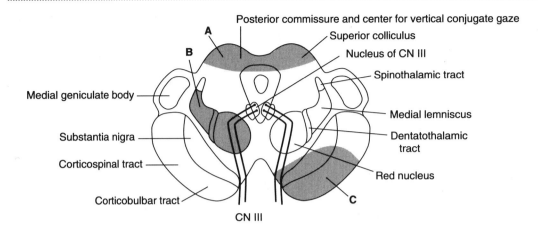

Figure 14-3. Lesions of the rostral midbrain at the level of the superior colliculus and oculomotor nucleus of CN III. (A) Dorsal midbrain (Parinaud) syndrome. (B) Paramedian midbrain (Benedikt) syndrome. (C) Medial midbrain (Weber) syndrome.

    C. Medial midbrain (Weber) syndrome (see Figure 14-3C). Affected structures and resultant deficits include:

        1. Oculomotor nerve roots (intra-axial fibers). Lesions here result in complete ipsilateral oculomotor paralysis; eye abduction and depression are due to intact lateral rectus (CN VI) and superior oblique (CN IV) muscles. Ptosis and an ipsilateral fixed and dilated pupil also occur.

        2. Corticospinal tracts. Lesions here result in contralateral spastic hemiparesis.

        3. Corticobulbar fibers. Lesions here result in contralateral weakness of the lower face (CN VII), tongue (CN XII), and palate (CN X). (The upper face division of the facial nucleus receives bilateral corticobulbar input.) The uvula and pharyngeal wall are pulled toward the normal side (CN X), and the protruded tongue points to the weak side.

IV. ACOUSTIC NEUROMA (schwannoma) is a benign tumor of Schwann cells that affects the vestibulocochlear nerve (CN VIII). It is a posterior fossa tumor of the internal auditory meatus and the cerebellopontine (CP) angle. Frequently, the neuroma compresses the facial nerve (CN VII), which accompanies CN VIII in the cerebellopontine angle and internal auditory meatus. It may impinge on the pons and affect the spinal trigeminal tract (CN V). This condition, which occurs in twice as many women as men, includes the following affected structures and resultant deficits:

    A. Cochlear nerve of CN VIII. Damage causes tinnitus and unilateral nerve deafness.

    B. Vestibular nerve of CN VIII. If this nerve is affected, vertigo, nystagmus, nausea, vomiting, and unsteadiness of gait occur.

    C. Facial nerve (CN VII). Facial weakness and loss of the corneal reflex (efferent limb) occur if the facial nerve is affected.

    D. Spinal trigeminal tract (CN V). Damage to this tract results in paresthesias and anesthesia of ipsilateral face, as well as loss of the corneal reflex (afferent limb).

15

Cerebellum

I. FUNCTION OF THE CEREBELLUM. The cerebellum has three primary functions: **maintenance of posture and balance, maintenance of muscle tone,** and the **coordination of voluntary motor activity.**

II. ANATOMY OF THE CEREBELLUM

   A. Cerebellar peduncles

      1. Superior cerebellar peduncle. This structure contains the major output from the cerebellum, the dentatothalamic tract, which terminates in the ventral lateral nucleus of the thalamus. It contains one major afferent pathway, the ventral superior cerebellar tract (VSCT).

      2. Middle cerebellar peduncle. This structure receives pontocerebellar fibers, which project to the neocerebellum (pontocerebellum).

      3. Inferior cerebellar peduncle. This structure contains three major afferent tracts: the dorsal spinal cerebellar tract (DSCT), the cuneocerebellar tract, and the olivocerebellar tract from the contralateral inferior olivary nucleus.

   B. Cerebellar cortex, neurons, and fibers

      1. Cerebellar cortex contains three layers.
         a. The **molecular layer** is the outer layer underlying the pia. It contains stellate cells, basket cells, and the dendritic arbor of the Purkinje cells.
         b. The **Purkinje cell layer** is found between the molecular and granule cell layers.
         c. The **granular layer** is the inner layer overlying the white matter. It contains granule cells, Golgi cells, and cerebellar glomeruli. A cerebellar glomerulus consists of a mossy fiber rosette, granule cell dendrites, and a Golgi cell axon.

      2. Neurons and fibers of the cerebellum
         a. Purkinje cells convey the only output from the cerebellar cortex. They project inhibitory output [i.e., γ-aminobutyric acid (GABA)] to the cerebellar and vestibular nuclei. They are excited by parallel and climbing fibers. They are inhibited by GABA-ergic basket and stellate cells.
         b. Granule cells excite (via glutamate) Purkinje, basket, stellate, and Golgi cells via parallel fibers. They are inhibited by Golgi cells and are excited by mossy fibers.
         c. Parallel fibers are the axons of granule cells that extend into the molecular layer.

d. Mossy fibers are the afferent excitatory fibers of the spinocerebellar, pontocerebellar, and vestibulocerebellar tracts. They terminate as mossy fiber rosettes on granule cell dendrites. They excite granule cells to discharge via their parallel fibers.

e. Climbing fibers are the afferent excitatory (via aspartate) fibers of the olivocerebellar tract. These fibers arise from the contralateral inferior olivary nucleus and terminate on neurons of the cerebellar nuclei and on dendrites of Purkinje cells.

III. MAJOR CEREBELLAR PATHWAY (Figure 15-1). This pathway consists of the following structures:

A. The **Purkinje cells of the cerebellar cortex** project to the cerebellar nuclei (e.g., dentate, emboliform, globose, and fastigial nuclei).

B. The **dentate nucleus** is the major effector nucleus of the cerebellum. It gives rise to the dentatothalamic tract, which projects via the superior cerebellar peduncle (SCP) to the contralateral ventral lateral (VL) nucleus of the thalamus. The decussation of the SCP is in the caudal midbrain tegmentum.

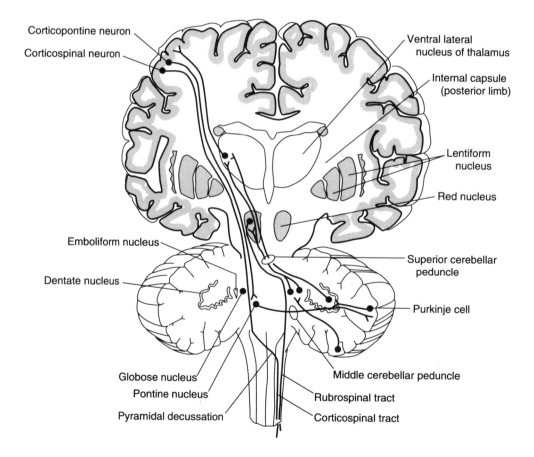

Figure 15-1. Principal cerebellar connections. The major efferent pathway is the dentatothalamocortical tract. The cerebellum receives input from the cerebral cortex via the corticopontocerebellar tract.

C. The **ventral lateral nucleus of the thalamus** receives the dentatothalamic tract. It projects to the primary motor cortex of the precentral gyrus (area 4).

D. The **motor cortex (motor strip or area 4)** receives input from the VL nucleus of the thalamus. It projects as the corticopontine tract to the pontine nuclei.

E. Pontine nuclei receive input from the motor cortex. Axons project as the pontocerebellar tract to the contralateral cerebellar cortex, where they terminate as mossy fibers, thus completing the circuit.

IV. CEREBELLAR DYSFUNCTION includes the following triad:

A. Hypotonia is a loss in the resistance normally offered by muscles to palpation or to passive manipulation. It results in a floppy, loose-jointed, rag-doll appearance with pendular reflexes; the patient appears inebriated.

B. Disequilibrium refers to the loss of balance, characterized by gait and trunk dystaxia.

C. Dyssynergia is a loss of coordinated muscle activity and includes **dysmetria, intention tremor, failure to check movements, nystagmus, dysdiadochokinesia, and dysrhythmokinesia.**

V. CEREBELLAR SYNDROMES AND TUMORS

A. Anterior vermis syndrome involves the leg region of the anterior lobe. It results from atrophy of the rostral vermis, most commonly caused by alcohol abuse. It results in gait, trunk, and leg dystaxia.

B. Posterior vermis syndrome involves the flocculonodular lobe. It is usually the result of brain tumors in children and is most commonly caused by medulloblastomas or ependymomas. This syndrome results in truncal dystaxia.

C. Hemispheric syndrome usually involves one cerebellar hemisphere. It is frequently the result of a brain tumor (astrocytoma) or an abscess (secondary to otitis media or mastoiditis). It results in arm, leg, and gait dystaxia and in cerebellar signs that are ipsilateral to the lesion.

D. Cerebellar tumors. In children, 70% of brain tumors are found in the posterior fossa.

    1. Astrocytomas constitute 30% of all brain tumors in children. They are most frequently found in the cerebellar hemisphere. After surgical removal, it is common for the child to survive for many years.

    2. Medulloblastomas are malignant and constitute 20% of all brain tumors in children. They are thought to originate from the superficial granule layer of the cerebellar cortex. They usually obstruct passage of cerebrospinal fluid (CSF), which causes hydrocephalus.

    3. Ependymomas constitute 15% of all brain tumors in children. They occur most frequently in the fourth ventricle. They usually obstruct CSF passage and cause hydrocephalus.

16

Thalamus

I. INTRODUCTION. The thalamus is the largest division of the diencephalon. It plays an important role in sensory and motor systems integration.

II. MAJOR THALAMIC NUCLEI AND THEIR CONNECTIONS (Figure 16-1)

A. The **anterior nucleus** receives hypothalamic input from the mamillary nucleus via the mamillothalamic tract. It projects to the cingulate gyrus. The anterior nucleus is part of the Papez circuit of emotion of the limbic system.

B. The **mediodorsal nucleus** (dorsomedial nucleus) is reciprocally connected to the prefrontal cortex. It has abundant connections with intralaminar nuclei. It receives input from the amygdala, the substantia nigra, and the temporal neocortex. When destroyed, **memory loss** occurs (Wernicke-Korsakoff syndrome). The mediodorsal nucleus plays a role in the expression of affect, emotion, and behavior (limbic function).

C. The **centromedian nucleus** is the largest of the intralaminar nuclei. It is reciprocally connected to the motor cortex (area 4). The centromedian nucleus receives input from the globus pallidus. It projects to the striatum (caudate nucleus and putamen) and projects diffusely to the entire neocortex.

D. The **pulvinar** is the largest thalamic nucleus. It has reciprocal connections with the association cortex of the occipital, parietal, and posterior temporal lobes. It receives input from the lateral and medial geniculate bodies and the superior colliculus. It is involved with the **integration of visual, auditory, and somesthetic input**. Destruction of the dominant pulvinar may result in sensory dysphasia.

E. Ventral tier nuclei

1. The **ventral anterior nucleus** receives input from the globus pallidus and the substantia nigra. It projects diffusely to the prefrontal and orbital cortices, and to the premotor cortex (area 6).

2. The **ventral lateral nucleus** receives input from the cerebellum (dentate nucleus), globus pallidus, and substantia nigra. It projects to the motor cortex (area 4) and to the supplementary motor cortex (area 6).

3. The **ventral posterior nucleus** (ventrobasal complex) is the nucleus of termination of general somatic afferent (GSA; touch, pain, and temperature) and special visceral afferent (SVA; taste) fibers. It contains two subnuclei:

a. The **ventral posterolateral (VPL) nucleus** receives the spinothalamic tracts and the medial lemniscus. It projects to the somesthetic (sensory) cortex (areas 3, 1, and 2).

A

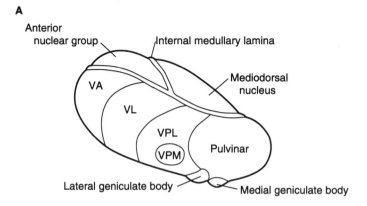

B

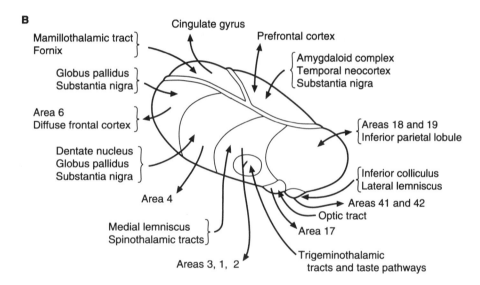

Figure 16-1. Major thalamic nuclei and their connections. (A) Dorsolateral aspect and major nuclei. (B) Major afferent and efferent connections. *VA* = ventral anterior nucleus; *VL* = ventral lateral nucleus; *VPL* = ventral posterior lateral nucleus; *VPM* = ventral posterior medial nucleus.

        b. The **ventral posteromedial (VPM) nucleus** receives the trigeminothalamic tracts. It receives the taste pathway from the solitary nucleus via the central tegmental tract. It projects to the somesthetic (sensory) cortex (areas 3, 1, and 2).

F. **Metathalamus**

    1. The **lateral geniculate body** is a visual relay nucleus. It receives retinal input via the optic tract. It projects to the primary visual cortex (area 17).

    2. The **medial geniculate body** is an auditory relay nucleus. It receives auditory input via the brachium of the inferior colliculus. It projects to the primary auditory cortex (areas 41 and 42).

III. BLOOD SUPPLY OF THE THALAMUS. The thalamus is irrigated by three arteries (see Chapter 3).

   A. Posterior communicating artery

   B. Posterior cerebral artery

   C. Anterior choroidal artery (lateral geniculate body)

IV. THE INTERNAL CAPSULE (Figure 16-2) is a layer of white matter (myelinated axons) that separate the caudate nucleus and the thalamus medially from the lentiform nucleus laterally.

   A. The **anterior limb** is located between the caudate nucleus and the lentiform nucleus (globus pallidus and the putamen).

   B. The **genu** contains the corticobulbar fibers.

   C. The **posterior limb** is located between the thalamus and the lentiform nucleus. It contains corticospinal (pyramidal) fibers. It also contains sensory radiations (pain, temperature, and touch) as well as the visual and auditory radiations.

   D. Blood supply of the internal capsule

      1. The **anterior limb** is irrigated by the medial striate branches of the anterior cerebral artery and by the lateral striate (lenticulostriate) branches of the middle cerebral artery.

      2. The **genu** is perfused either by direct branches from the internal carotid artery or by the pallidal branches of the anterior choroidal artery.

      3. The **posterior limb** is supplied by branches of the anterior choroidal artery and lenticulostriate branches of the middle cerebral arteries.

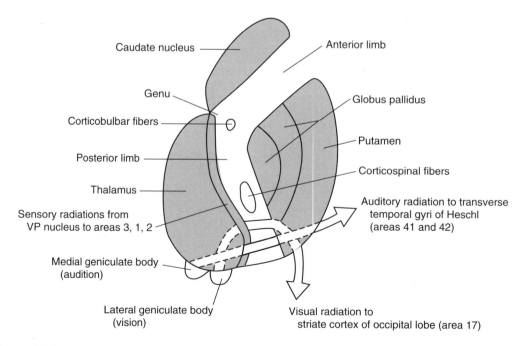

Figure 16-2. Horizontal section of the right internal capsule showing the major fiber projections. Clinically important tracts lie in the genu and in the posterior limb. Lesions of the internal capsule result in contralateral hemiparesis and contralateral hemianopia.

17

Visual System

I. **INTRODUCTION.** The visual system is served by the optic nerve, which is a special somatic afferent (SSA) nerve.

II. **THE VISUAL PATHWAY** (Figure 17-1) consists of the following structures:

   A. **Ganglion cells of the retina** form the optic nerve, CN II. They project from the nasal hemiretina to the contralateral lateral geniculate body and from the temporal hemiretina to the ipsilateral lateral geniculate body.

   B. The **optic nerve** projects from the lamina cribrosa of the scleral canal and via the optic canal to the optic chiasm.

   1. **Transection of the optic nerve** results in ipsilateral blindness, and no direct pupillary light reflex.

   2. The section of the optic nerve at the optic chiasm transects all fibers from the ipsilateral retina and fibers from the contralateral inferior nasal quadrant that loop into the optic nerve; this **lesion** results in a blind eye on the side of transection and an upper temporal quadrant defect in the contralateral eye (**junction scotoma**).

   C. The **optic chiasm** contains decussating fibers from the two nasal hemiretinae. It contains noncrossing fibers from the two temporal hemiretinae and projects fibers to the suprachiasmatic nucleus of the hypothalamus.

   1. **Midsagittal transection or pressure** (frequently from a pituitary tumor) results in bitemporal hemianopia.

   2. **Bilateral lateral compression** results in binasal hemianopia (calcified internal carotid arteries).

   D. The **optic tract** contains fibers from the ipsilateral temporal hemiretina and the contralateral nasal hemiretina. It projects to the ipsilateral lateral geniculate body, the pretectal nuclei, and the superior colliculus. Transection results in a contralateral hemianopia.

   E. The **lateral geniculate body** is a six-layered nucleus; layers 1, 4, and 6 receive crossed fibers; layers 2, 3, and 5 receive uncrossed fibers. The lateral geniculate body receives input from layer VI of the striate cortex (area 17) and receives fibers from the ipsilateral temporal hemiretina and the contralateral nasal hemiretina. It projects, via the geniculocalcarine tract, to the primary visual cortex (area 17).

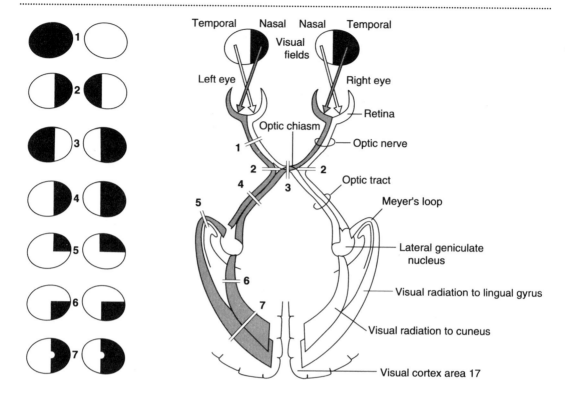

Figure 17-1. Visual pathway from the retina to the visual cortex showing visual field defects: (*1*) Total blindness in left eye; (*2*) Binasal hemianopia; (*3*) Bitemporal hemianopia; (*4*) Right hemianopia; (*5*) Right upper quadrantanopia; (*6*) Right lower quadrantanopia; (*7*) Right hemianopia with macular sparing.

F. The **geniculocalcarine tract (visual radiation)** projects via two divisions to the visual cortex:

    1. The **upper division** (see Figure 17-1) projects to the upper bank of the calcarine sulcus, the cuneus. It contains input from superior retinal quadrants, representing inferior visual field quadrants.

        a. Transection results in a contralateral lower quadrantanopia.

        b. Lesions involving both cunei result in a lower altitudinal hemianopia (altitudinopia).

    2. The **lower division** (see Figure 17-1) loops from the lateral geniculate body anteriorly (Meyer's loop), then posteriorly to terminate in the lower bank of the calcarine sulcus, the lingual gyrus. It contains input from inferior retinal quadrants, representing superior visual field quadrants.

        a. Transection results in a **contralateral upper quadrantanopia** ("pie in the sky").

        b. Transection of both lingual gyri results in an **upper altitudinal hemianopia (altitudinopia)**.

G. The **visual cortex (area 17)** is found on the banks of the calcarine fissure. The **cuneus** is the upper bank. The **lingual gyrus** is the lower bank. Lesions result in a **contralateral hemianopia** with macular sparing. The visual cortex has a **retinotopic organization**:

    1. The **posterior area** receives macular input (central vision).

2. The **intermediate area** receives paramacular input (peripheral input).

3. The **anterior area** receives monocular input.

III. THE PUPILLARY LIGHT REFLEX PATHWAY (Figure 17-2) comprises an afferent limb, CN II, and an efferent limb, CN III. It consists of the following structures:

A. **Ganglion cells of the retina** project bilaterally to the pretectal nuclei.

B. The **pretectal nucleus of the midbrain** projects (via the posterior commissure) crossed and uncrossed fibers to the Edinger-Westphal nucleus.

C. The **Edinger-Westphal nucleus of CN III** gives rise to preganglionic parasympathetic fibers, which exit the midbrain with CN III and synapse with postganglionic parasympathetic neurons of the ciliary ganglion.

D. The **ciliary ganglion** gives rise to postganglionic parasympathetic fibers, which innervate the sphincter muscle of the iris.

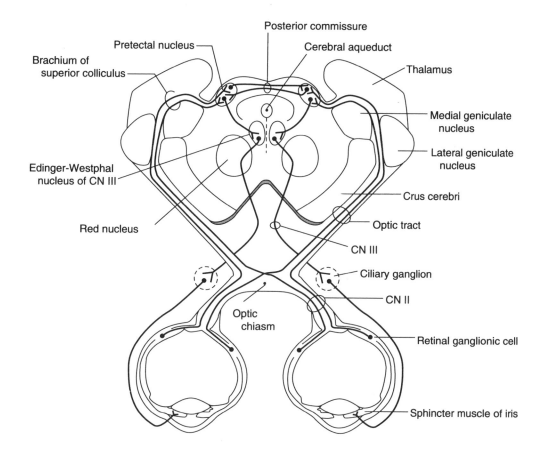

Figure 17-2. Diagram of the pupillary light pathway. Light shined into one eye causes both pupils to constrict. The response in the stimulated eye is called the direct pupillary light reflex; the response in the opposite eye is called the consensual pupillary light reflex.

IV. THE PUPILLARY DILATION PATHWAY (see Figure 7-5) is mediated by the sympathetic division of the autonomic nervous system. Interruption at any level results in an ipsilateral Horner's syndrome. This pathway consists of the following structures:

   A. Hypothalamus. Hypothalamic neurons project directly to the ciliospinal center (T1-T2) of the intermediolateral cell column.

   B. The **ciliospinal center of Budge (T1-T2)** projects preganglionic sympathetic fibers via the sympathetic trunk to the superior cervical ganglion.

   C. The **superior cervical ganglion** projects postganglionic sympathetic fibers via the perivascular plexus of the carotid system to the dilator muscle of the iris. Postganglionic sympathetic fibers pass through the **tympanic cavity** and **cavernous sinus** and enter the orbit via the **superior orbital fissure**.

V. NEAR REFLEX AND ACCOMMODATION PATHWAY

   A. The **cortical visual pathway** projects from the primary visual cortex (area 17) to the visual association cortex (area 19).

   B. The **visual association cortex (area 19)** projects via the corticotectal tract to the superior colliculus and pretectal nucleus.

   C. The **superior colliculus and pretectal nucleus** project to the **oculomotor complex of the midbrain:**

      1. The **rostral Edinger-Westphal nucleus** mediates pupillary constriction via the ciliary ganglion.

      2. The **caudal Edinger-Westphal nucleus** mediates contraction of the ciliary muscle, resulting in an increase in refractive power of the lens.

      3. The **medial rectus subnucleus of CN III** mediates convergence.

VI. CORTICAL AND SUBCORTICAL CENTERS FOR OCULAR MOTILITY

   A. The **frontal eye field** is located in the posterior part of the middle frontal gyrus (area 8). It is a center for voluntary (saccadic) eye movements.

      1. Stimulation (e.g., from an irritative lesion) results in **contralateral deviation of the eyes** (i.e., away from the lesion).

      2. Destruction results in **transient ipsilateral conjugate deviation of the eyes** toward the lesion.

   B. Occipital eye fields are located in areas 18 and 19 of the occipital lobes. These fields are cortical centers for involuntary (smooth) pursuit and tracking movements. **Stimulation** results in contralateral conjugate deviation of the eyes.

   C. The **subcortical center for lateral conjugate gaze** is located in the abducent nucleus of the pons (Figure 17-3). Some authorities place this "center" in the paramedian pontine reticular formation (PPRF).

      1. It receives input from the contralateral frontal eyefield.

      2. It projects to the ipsilateral lateral rectus muscle and, via the medial longitudinal fasciculus (MLF), to the contralateral medial rectus subnucleus of the oculomotor complex.

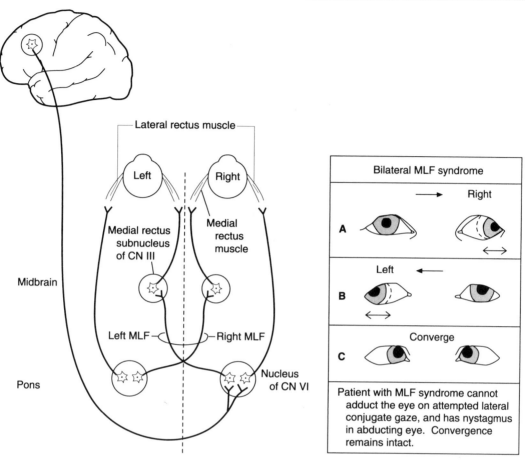

Figure 17-3. Connections of the pontine center for lateral conjugate gaze. Lesions of the medial longitudinal fasciculus (MLF) between the abducent and oculomotor nuclei result in a medial rectus palsy on attempted lateral conjugate gaze and horizontal nystagmus in the abducting eye. Convergence remains intact (see *inset*). A unilateral MLF lesion would affect the ipsilateral medial rectus only.

    D. The **subcortical center for vertical conjugate gaze** is located in the midbrain at the level of the posterior commissure. It is called the rostral interstitial nucleus of the MLF (riMLF) and is associated with **Parinaud's syndrome** (see Figure 14-3A).

VII. CLINICAL CORRELATIONS

    A. **MLF syndrome** (see Figure 17-3) is a condition in which there is damage (demyelination) to the MLF between the abducent and oculomotor nuclei. It results in **medial rectus palsy** on attempted lateral conjugate gaze and **monocular horizontal nystagmus** in the abducting eye (**convergence is normal**). This syndrome is most commonly seen in patients with **multiple sclerosis**.

    B. **Argyll Robertson pupil** (pupillary light–near dissociation) is the absence of a miotic reaction to light, both direct and consensual, with the preservation of a miotic reaction to near stimulus (accommodation–convergence). It may be present in **syphilis** and **diabetes**.

C. Horner's syndrome results from transection of the oculosympathetic pathway at any level (see IV). This syndrome consists of miosis, ptosis, apparent enophthalmos, and hemianhidrosis.

D. Transtentorial herniation (uncal herniation) occurs as the result of **increased supratentorial pressure,** which is commonly due to a brain tumor or a hematoma (subdural or epidural).

1. The pressure cone forces the parahippocampal uncus through the tentorial incisure.

2. The impacted uncus forces the contralateral crus cerebri against the tentorial edge (Kernohan notch) and puts pressure on the ipsilateral CN III and the posterior cerebral artery, resulting in the following neurologic deficits:

   a. Ipsilateral hemiparesis due to pressure on the corticospinal tract located in the contralateral crus cerebri

   b. A fixed and dilated pupil, ptosis, and a "down-and-out" eye, which are due to pressure on the ipsilateral oculomotor nerve

   c. Contralateral homonymous hemianopia caused by compression of the posterior cerebral artery, which irrigates the visual cortex

E. Papilledema (choked disk) is a noninflammatory congestion of the optic disk caused by increased intracranial pressure. It is most commonly caused by brain tumors, subdural hematoma, and hydrocephalus. It usually **does not alter visual acuity;** it may result in bilateral **increased blind spots.** It is frequently asymmetric and will be greater on the side of the supratentorial lesion.

18

Autonomic Nervous System

I. **INTRODUCTION.** The autonomic nervous system (ANS) is a general visceral efferent (GVE) motor system that **controls and regulates smooth muscle, cardiac muscle, and glands.**

   A. The ANS consists of two types of **projection neurons:**

      1. **Preganglionic neurons**

      2. **Postganglionic neurons** (sympathetic ganglia have interneurons)

   B. **Autonomic output** is controlled by the **hypothalamus.**

   C. The ANS has **three divisions:**

      1. **Sympathetic.** Figure 18-1 shows sympathetic innervation of the ANS.

      2. **Parasympathetic.** Figure 18-2 details the parasympathetic innervation of the ANS. Sympathetic and parasympathetic activity on organ systems is compared in Table 18-1.

      3. **Enteric.** The enteric division includes the intramural ganglia of the gastrointestinal tract, the submucosal plexus and the myenteric plexus.

II. **CRANIAL NERVES WITH PARASYMPATHETIC COMPONENTS** include the following:

   A. **CN III,** ciliary ganglion

   B. **CN VII,** pterygopalatine and submandibular ganglia

   C. **CN IX,** otic ganglion

   D. **CN X,** terminal (mural) ganglia

III. **COMMUNICATING RAMI** of the ANS

   A. **White communicating rami** are found between T-1 and L-3.

   B. **Gray communicating rami** are found at all spinal levels.

IV. **NEUROTRANSMITTERS** of the ANS include:

   A. **Acetylcholine (ACh),** which is the neurotransmitter of preganglionic neurons

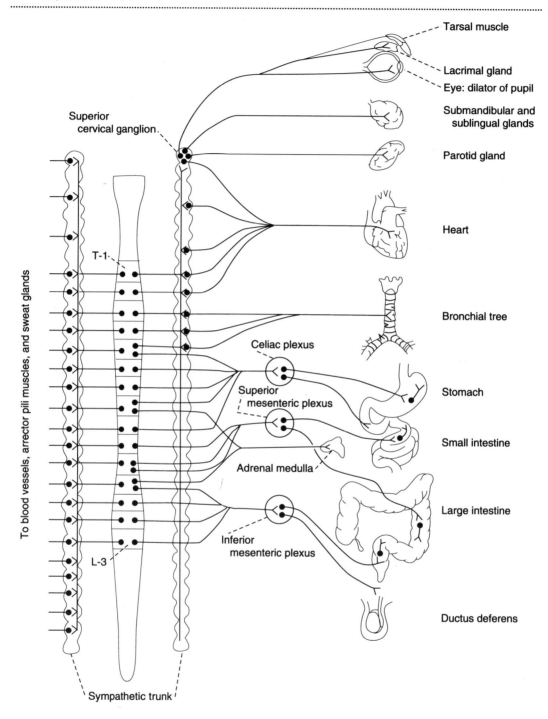

Figure 18-1. Schematic diagram showing the sympathetic (thoracolumbar) innervation of the autonomic nervous system (ANS). Note that the entire sympathetic innervation of the head is via the superior cervical ganglion. Gray communicating rami are found at all spinal cord levels; white communicating rami are found only in spinal segments T1-L3.

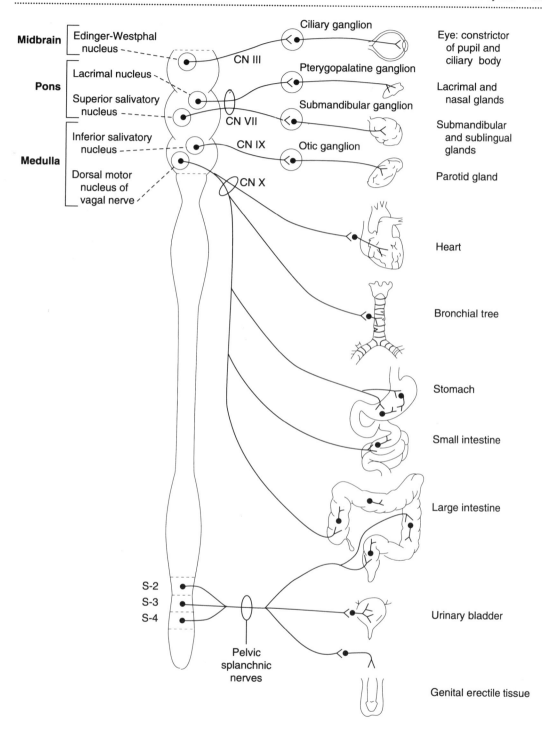

Figure 18-2. Schematic diagram showing the parasympathetic (craniosacral) innervation of the autonomic nervous system (ANS). Sacral outflow includes segments S2-S4. Cranial outflow is mediated via four cranial nerves: CN III, CN VII, CN IX, and CN X.

Table 18-1
Sympathetic and Parasympathetic Activity on Organ Systems

Structure	Sympathetic Function	Parasympathetic Function
Eye		
Radial muscle of iris	Dilates pupil (mydriasis)	
Circular muscle of iris		Constricts pupil (miosis)
Ciliary muscle of ciliary body		Contracts for near vision
Lacrimal gland		Stimulates secretion
Salivary glands	Viscous secretion	Watery secretion
Sweat glands		
Thermoregulatory	Increases	
Apocrine (stress)	Increases	
Heart		
Sinoatrial node	Accelerates	Decelerates (vagal arrest)
Atrioventricular node	Increases conduction velocity	Decreases conduction velocity
Contractility	Increases	Decreases (atria)
Vascular smooth muscle		
Skin, splanchnic vessels	Contracts	
Skeletal muscle vessels	Relaxes	
Bronchiolar smooth muscle	Relaxes	Contracts
Gastrointestinal tract		
Smooth muscle		
Walls	Relaxes	Contracts
Sphincters	Contracts	Relaxes
Secretion and motility	Decreases	Increases
Genitourinary tract		
Smooth muscle		
Bladder wall	Little or no effect	Contracts
Sphincter	Contracts	Relaxes
Penis, seminal vesicles	Ejaculation	Erection
Adrenal medulla	Secretes epinephrine and norepinephrine	
Metabolic functions		
Liver	Gluconeogenesis and glycogenolysis	
Fat cells	Lipolysis	
Kidney	Renin release	

Reprinted with permission from Fix J: *BRS Neuroanatomy,* Media, William & Wilkins, 1991.

B. Norepinephrine, which is the neurotransmitter of postganglionic neurons, with the exception of sweat glands and some blood vessels that receive cholinergic sympathetic innervation

C. Dopamine, which is the neurotransmitter of the small intensely fluorescent (SIF) cells, which are interneurons of the sympathetic ganglia

D. Vasoactive intestinal polypeptide (VIP) is co-localized with ACh in some postganglionic parasympathetic fibers. It is a vasodilator.

E. **Nitric oxide (NO)** is a newly discovered neurotransmitter that is responsible for relaxation of smooth muscle. It is responsible for penile erection (see Chapter 22).

V. CLINICAL CORRELATIONS

A. **Megacolon (Hirschsprung's disease)** is also called congenital aganglionic megacolon. It is characterized by extreme dilation and hypertrophy of the colon with fecal retention and by the absence of ganglion cells in the myenteric plexus. It results from the failure of neural crest cells to migrate into the colon.

B. **Familial dysautonomia (Riley-Day syndrome)** affects Jewish children predominantly. It is an autosomal recessive trait characterized by abnormal sweating, blood pressure instability (e.g., orthostatic hypotension), difficulty in feeding due to inadequate muscle tone in the gastrointestinal tract, and progressive sensory loss. It results in the loss of neurons in autonomic and sensory ganglia.

C. **Raynaud's disease** is a painful disorder of the terminal arteries of the extremities. It is characterized by idiopathic paroxysmal bilateral cyanosis of the digits, due to arterial and arteriolar constriction caused by cold or emotion. It may be treated by preganglionic sympathectomy.

D. **Peptic ulcer disease** results from excessive production of hydrochloric acid because of increased parasympathetic (tone) stimulation.

E. **Horner's syndrome** (see Chapter 17) is oculosympathetic paralysis.

F. **Shy-Drager syndrome** involves preganglionic sympathetic neurons from the intermediolateral cell column. It is characterized by orthostatic hypotension, anhidrosis, impotence, and bladder atonicity.

G. **Botulism.** The toxin of *Clostridium botulinum* blocks the release of ACh and results in paralysis of all striated muscles. Autonomic effects include dry eyes, dry mouth, and gastrointestinal ileus (bowel obstruction).

19

Hypothalamus

I. INTRODUCTION

A. General structure and function. The hypothalamus is a **division of the diencephalon** that subserves three systems: the autonomic nervous system, the endocrine system, and the limbic system. It functions in the maintenance of homeostasis.

B. Major hypothalamic nuclei and their functions

1. The **medial preoptic nucleus** (Figure 19-1) regulates the release of gonadotropic hormones from the adenohypophysis. It contains the sexually dimorphic nucleus, the development of which depends on testosterone levels.

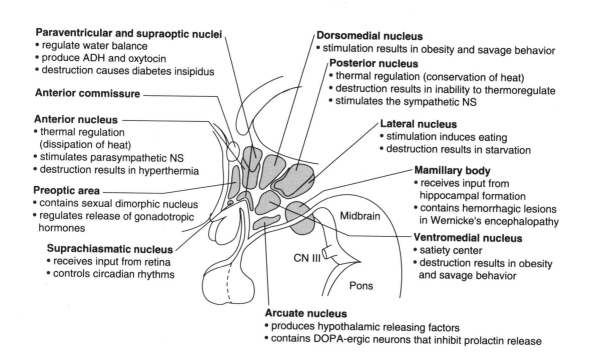

Paraventricular and supraoptic nuclei
• regulate water balance
• produce ADH and oxytocin
• destruction causes diabetes insipidus

Anterior commissure

Anterior nucleus
• thermal regulation
  (dissipation of heat)
• stimulates parasympathetic NS
• destruction results in hyperthermia

Preoptic area
• contains sexual dimorphic nucleus
• regulates release of gonadotropic
  hormones

Suprachiasmatic nucleus
• receives input from retina
• controls circadian rhythms

Dorsomedial nucleus
• stimulation results in obesity and savage behavior

Posterior nucleus
• thermal regulation (conservation of heat)
• destruction results in inability to thermoregulate
• stimulates the sympathetic NS

Lateral nucleus
• stimulation induces eating
• destruction results in starvation

Mamillary body
• receives input from
  hippocampal formation
• contains hemorrhagic lesions
  in Wernicke's encephalopathy

Ventromedial nucleus
• satiety center
• destruction results in obesity
  and savage behavior

Midbrain

CN III

Pons

Arcuate nucleus
• produces hypothalamic releasing factors
• contains DOPA-ergic neurons that inhibit prolactin release

Figure 19-1. Major hypothalamic nuclei and their functions.

2. The **suprachiasmatic nucleus** receives direct input from the retina. It plays a role in the regulation of circadian rhythms.

3. The **anterior nucleus** plays a role in temperature regulation. It stimulates the parasympathetic nervous system. Destruction of this nucleus results in hyperthermia.

4. The **paraventricular nucleus** (Figure 19-2) synthesizes antidiuretic hormone (ADH), oxytocin, and corticotropin-releasing hormone (CRH). It gives rise to the supraopticohypophyseal tract, which projects to the neurohypophysis. It regulates water balance (conservation of water). Destruction results in diabetes insipidus.

5. The **supraoptic nucleus** synthesizes ADH and oxytocin in a manner similar to that of the paraventricular nucleus.

6. The **dorsomedial nucleus.** Savage behavior results when this nucleus is stimulated in animals.

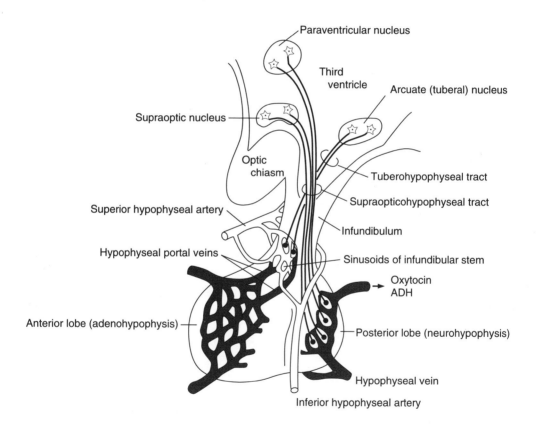

Figure 19-2. The hypophyseal portal system. The paraventricular and supraoptic nuclei produce antidiuretic hormone (ADH) and oxytocin and transport the substances via the supraopticohypophyseal tract to the capillary bed of the neurohypophysis. The arcuate nucleus of the infundibulum transports releasing hormones via the tuberohypophyseal tract to the sinusoids of the infundibular stem, which drain into the secondary capillary plexus in the adenohypophysis.

7. The **ventromedial nucleus** is considered a satiety center. When stimulated, it inhibits the urge to eat. Bilateral destruction results in hyperphagia, obesity, and savage behavior.

8. The **arcuate (infundibular) nucleus** contains neurons that produce hypothalamic-releasing/inhibiting factors and gives rise to the tuberohypophyseal tract, which terminates in the hypophyseal portal system (see Figure 19-2) of the infundibulum (medium eminence). The arcuate nucleus contains neurons that produce dopamine [i.e., prolactin-inhibiting factor (PIF)].

9. The **mamillary nucleus** receives input from the hippocampal formation via the (postcommissural) fornix. It projects to the anterior nucleus of the thalamus via the mamillothalamic tract (part of Papez circuit). Patients with Wernicke's encephalopathy, which is a thiamine (vitamin B_1) deficiency, have lesions in the mamillary nucleus. Lesions here are also associated with alcoholism.

10. The **posterior hypothalamic nucleus** plays a role in thermal regulation (i.e., conservation and increased production of heat). Lesions here result in **poikilothermia**, which is the inability to thermoregulate.

11. The **lateral hypothalamic nucleus** induces eating when stimulated. **Lesions** in this nucleus cause **anorexia and starvation**.

C. Major fiber systems of the hypothalamus

1. The **fornix** is the largest projection to the hypothalamus. It projects from the hippocampal formation to the mamillary nucleus, anterior nucleus of the thalamus, and the septal area. It projects from the septal area to the hippocampal formation.

2. The **medial forebrain bundle** traverses the entire lateral hypothalamic area. It interconnects the orbitofrontal cortex, septal area, hypothalamus, and the midbrain.

3. The **mamillothalamic tract** projects from the mamillary nuclei to the anterior nucleus of the thalamus (part of Papez circuit).

4. The **stria terminalis** is the major pathway from the amygdala. It interconnects the septal area, the hypothalamus, and the amygdala.

5. The **supraopticohypophysial tract** conducts fibers from the supraoptic and paraventricular nuclei to the neurohypophysis, which is the release site for ADH and oxytocin.

6. The **tuberohypophysial (tuberoinfundibular) tract** conducts fibers from the arcuate nucleus to the hypophyseal portal system (see Figure 19-2).

7. The **hypothalamospinal tract** contains direct descending autonomic fibers that influence preganglionic sympathetic neurons of the intermediolateral cell column and preganglionic neurons of the sacral parasympathetic nucleus. Interruption above the first thoracic segment (T-1) results in Horner's syndrome.

II. FUNCTIONS OF THE HYPOTHALAMUS

A. Autonomic function

1. The **anterior hypothalamus** has an excitatory effect on the parasympathetic nervous system.

2. The **posterior hypothalamus** has an excitatory effect on the sympathetic nervous system.

B. **Temperature regulation**

    1. The **anterior hypothalamus** regulates and maintains body temperature. Destruction of this area causes hyperthermia.

    2. The **posterior hypothalamus** helps produce and conserve heat. Destruction of this area causes the inability to thermoregulate.

C. **Water balance regulation.** The **paraventricular nucleus** synthesizes antidiuretic hormone (ADH), which controls water excretion by the kidneys.

D. **Food intake regulation.** Two hypothalamic nuclei play roles in the control of appetite.

    1. When stimulated, the **ventromedial nucleus** inhibits the urge to eat. Bilateral destruction results in hyperphagia, obesity, and savage behavior.

    2. When stimulated, the **lateral hypothalamic nucleus** induces the urge to eat. Destruction of this area causes starvation and emaciation.

III. CLINICAL CORRELATIONS

A. **Diabetes insipidus,** which is characterized by polyuria and polydipsia, is the best known of the hypothalamic syndromes. It results from lesions of the ADH pathways to the posterior lobe of the pituitary gland.

B. **Syndrome of inappropriate ADH secretion (SIADH)** is usually caused by lung tumors or by drug therapy (e.g., carbamazepine or chlorpromazine).

C. **Craniopharyngioma** is a congenital tumor originating from remnants of Rathke's pouch (see Chapter 4) that is usually calcified. It is the most common supratentorial tumor found in children, and it is the most common cause of hypopituitarism in children.

    1. **Pressure on the chiasma** results in bitemporal hemianopia.

    2. **Pressure on the hypothalamus** causes the hypothalamic syndrome with adiposity, diabetes insipidus, disturbance of temperature regulation, and somnolence.

D. **Pituitary adenomas** constitute 15% of cases of clinical symptomatic intracranial tumors. They are rarely seen in children. When pituitary adenomas are endocrine-active, they produce endocrine abnormalities (e.g., amenorrhea and galactorrhea from a prolactin-secreting adenoma, the most common type).

    1. **Pressure on the chiasm** results in a bitemporal hemianopia.

    2. **Pressure on the hypothalamus** may cause the hypothalamus syndrome.

20

Limbic System

I. INTRODUCTION. The limbic system is considered to be the anatomic substrate underlying behavioral and emotional expression. It expresses itself through the hypothalamus via the autonomic nervous system.

II. MAJOR COMPONENTS AND CONNECTIONS

A. The **orbitofrontal cortex** mediates the conscious perception of smell. It has reciprocal connections with the mediodorsal nucleus of the thalamus. It is interconnected via the medial forebrain bundle with the septal area and the hypothalamic nuclei.

B. The **mediodorsal nucleus of the thalamus** has reciprocal connections with the orbitofrontal and prefrontal cortices and the hypothalamus. It receives input from the amygdala. It plays a role in affective behavior and memory.

C. The **anterior nucleus of the thalamus** receives input from the mamillary nucleus via the mamillothalamic tract and fornix. It projects to the cingulate gyrus and is a major link in the Papez circuit.

D. The **septal area** is a telencephalic structure. It has reciprocal connections with the hippocampal formation via the fornix, and it has reciprocal connections with the hypothalamus via the medial forebrain bundle. It projects via the stria medullaris (thalami) to the habenular nucleus.

E. The **limbic lobe** includes the subcallosal area, the paraterminal gyrus, the cingulate gyrus and isthmus, and the parahippocampal gyrus, which includes the uncus. It contains, buried in the parahippocampal gyrus, the hippocampal formation and the amygdaloid nuclear complex.

F. The **hippocampal formation** consists of a sheet of archicortex jelly-rolled into the parahippocampal gyrus. It functions in learning, memory, and recognition of novelty. It receives major input via the entorhinal cortex and projects major output via the fornix. **Major structures of the hippocampal formation** include the following.

1. The **dentate gyrus** has a three-layered archicortex. It contains granule cells that receive hippocampal input and project output to the pyramidal cells of the hippocampus and subiculum.

2. The **hippocampus (cornu Ammonis)** has a three-layered archicortex. It contains pyramidal cells that project via the fornix to the septal area and to the hypothalamus.

3. The **subiculum** receives input via the hippocampal pyramidal cells. It projects via the fornix to the mamillary nuclei and the anterior nucleus of the thalamus.

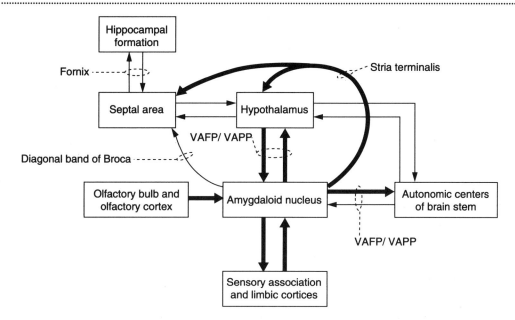

Figure 20-1. Major connections of the amygdaloid nucleus. The amygdaloid nucleus receives input from three major sources: the olfactory system, the sensory association and limbic cortices, and the hypothalamus. The major output from the amygdaloid nucleus is via two channels: The stria terminalis projects to the hypothalamus and the septal area, and the ventral amygdalofugal pathway (VAFP) projects to the hypothalamus, brain stem, and spinal cord. A smaller efferent bundle, the diagonal band of Broca, projects to the septal area. Afferent fibers from the hypothalamus and brain stem enter the amygdaloid nucleus via the ventral amygdalopetal pathway (VAPP).

> **G.** The **amygdaloid complex (amygdala)** [Figure 20-1; see also Figure 21-1] is a basal ganglion underlying the parahippocampal uncus. In humans, stimulation of the amygdala results in fear and signs of sympathetic overactivity. In other animals, stimulation results in cessation of activity and a heightened attentiveness. Lesions result in placidity and hypersexual behavior.
>
> > **1.** **Input** is from sensory association cortices, olfactory bulb and cortex, the hypothalamus and septal area, and the hippocampal formation.
> >
> > **2.** **Output** via the stria terminalis goes to the hypothalamus and the septal area. There is also output to the mediodorsal nucleus of the thalamus.
>
> **H.** The **hypothalamus** has reciprocal connections with the amygdala.
>
> **I.** The **limbic midbrain nuclei and associated neurotransmitters** include the ventral tegmental area (dopamine), raphe nuclei (serotonin), and the locus ceruleus (norepinephrine).

III. The Papez circuit (Figure 20-2) includes the following limbic structures.

> **A.** The **hippocampal formation** projects via the fornix to the mamillary nucleus and to the septal area.
>
> **B.** **Mamillary nucleus**
>
> **C.** **Anterior thalamic nucleus**

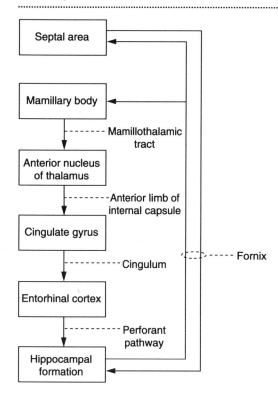

Figure 20-2. Major afferent and efferent limbic connections of the hippocampal formation. The hippocampal formation consists of three components: the hippocampus per se (cornu Ammonis), the subiculum, and the dentate gyrus. The hippocampus projects to the septal area; the subiculum projects to the mamillary nuclei; and the dentate gyrus does not project beyond the hippocampal formation. The circuit of Papez follows this route: hippocampal formation to mamillary nucleus to anterior thalamic nucleus to cingulate gyrus to entorhinal cortex to hippocampal formation.

   D. **Cingulate gyrus** (areas 24 and 23)

   E. **Entorhinal area** (area 28)

IV. CLINICAL CORRELATIONS

   A. **Klüver-Bucy syndrome** results from bilateral ablation of the anterior temporal lobes including the amygdaloid nuclei. It results in psychic blindness (visual agnosia), hyperphagia, docility (placidity), and hypersexuality.

   B. **The amnestic (confabulatory) syndrome** results from bilateral infarction of the hippocampal formation (i.e., hippocampal branches of the posterior cerebral arteries and the anterior choroidal arteries of the internal carotid arteries). It results in anterograde amnesia, which is an inability to learn and retain new information. **Memory loss should be associated with hippocampal pathology.**

21

Basal Ganglia and Striatal Motor System

I. BASAL GANGLIA (Figure 21-1)

   A. Components

      1. Caudate nucleus

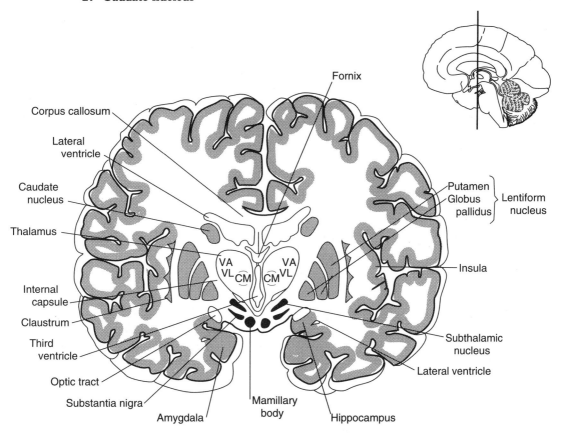

Figure 21-1. A coronal section through the midthalamus at the level of the mamillary bodies. The basal ganglia are all prominent at this level and include the striatum and the lentiform nucleus. The subthalamic nucleus and substantia nigra are important components of the striatal motor system.

  2. Putamen

  3. Globus pallidus

 B. Grouping of the basal ganglia

  1. The **striatum** consists of the caudate nucleus and putamen.

  2. The **lentiform nucleus** consists of the globus pallidus and putamen.

  3. The **corpus striatum** consists of the lentiform nucleus and the caudate nucleus.

II. STRIATAL (EXTRAPYRAMIDAL) MOTOR SYSTEM (see Figure 21-1). The striatal motor system plays a role in the initiation and execution of somatic motor activity, especially willed movement. It is involved in automatic stereotyped motor activity of a postural and reflex nature.

 A. **Structure.** The striatal motor system includes the following structures:

  1. Neocortex

  2. Striatum (caudatoputamen or neostriatum)

  3. Globus pallidus

  4. Subthalamic nucleus

  5. Substantia nigra (i.e., pars compacta and pars reticularis)

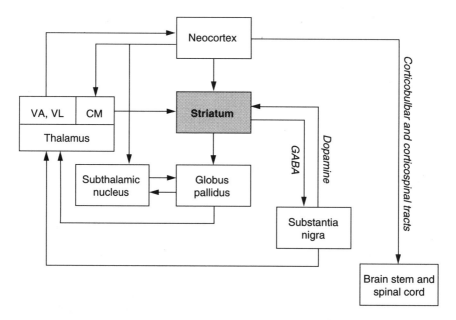

Figure 21-2. Major afferent and efferent connections of the striatal system. The striatum receives major input from three sources: the thalamus, the neocortex, and the substantia nigra. The striatum projects to the globus pallidus and the substantia nigra. The globus pallidus is the effector nucleus of the striatal system; it projects to the thalamus and to the subthalamic nucleus. The substantia nigra also projects to the thalamus. The striatal motor system expresses itself via the corticobulbar and corticospinal tracts. CM = centromedian nucleus; GABA = γ-aminobutyric acid; VA= ventral anterior nucleus; VL= ventral lateral nucleus.

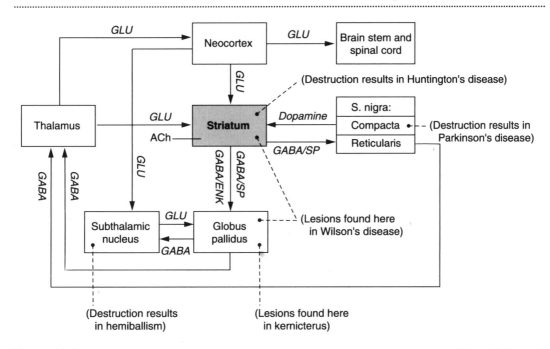

Figure 21-3. Major neurotransmitters of the striatal motor system. Within the striatum, globus pallidus, and pars reticularis of the substantia nigra, γ-aminobutyric acid (GABA) is the predominant neurotransmitter. GABA may coexist in the same neuron with enkephalin or substance P. Dopamine-containing neurons are found in the pars compacta of the substantia nigra. Acetylcholine is found in local circuit neurons of the striatum. The subthalamic nucleus projects excitatory glutaminergic fibers to the globus pallidus. ACh = acetylcholine; ENK = enkephalin; GLU = glutamate; SP = substance P.

     6. Thalamus [ventral anterior (VA), ventral lateral (VL), and centromedian (CM) nuclei]

  B. Figure 21-2 shows the **major afferent and efferent connections** of the striatal system.

  C. Neurotransmitters of the striatal system (Figure 21-3)

III. CLINICAL CORRELATIONS

  A. Parkinson's disease is a **degenerative disease** affecting the substantia nigra and its projections to the striatum.

    1. Results. Parkinson's disease results in the **depletion of dopamine** in the substantia nigra and striatum. It also results in a **loss of melanin-containing dopaminergic neurons** in the substantia nigra.

    2. Clinical signs are bradykinesia, stooped posture, shuffling gait, cogwheel rigidity, pill-rolling tremor, and masked facies. **Lewy bodies** are found in melanin-containing neurons of the substantia nigra.

  B. MPTP-induced parkinsonism. MPTP (methylphenyltetrahydropyridine) is an analog of meperidine (Demerol) that destroys dopaminergic neurons in the substantia nigra.

  C. Huntington's disease (Huntington's chorea) is an **inherited autosomal dominant movement disorder** that can be traced to a single gene defect on chromosome 4.

    1. The disease is associated with **degeneration of the cholinergic and γ-aminobutyric acid (GABA)-ergic neurons** of the striatum. It is accompanied by gyral atrophy in the frontal and temporal lobes.

    2. **Clinical signs** are choreiform movements, hypotonia, and progressive dementia.

D. **Other choreiform dyskinesias**

    1. **Sydenham's chorea (St. Vitus' dance)** is the most common cause of chorea overall. It is found mainly in girls, and occurs after a bout of rheumatic fever.

    2. **Chorea gravidarum** occurs usually during the second trimester of pregnancy. In many of these patients, a history of Sydenham's chorea can be obtained.

E. **Hemiballism** is a **movement disorder** usually resulting from a vascular lesion of the subthalamic nucleus. Clinical signs are violent contralateral **flinging (ballistic) movements of one or both extremities.**

F. **Hepatolenticular degeneration** (Wilson's disease) is an **autosomal recessive disorder** caused by a defect in the **metabolism of copper.** The gene locus is on chromosome 13.

    1. **Clinical signs** are choreiform or athetotic movements, rigidity, and **wing-beating tremor.**

    2. **Lesions** are found in the **lentiform nucleus.** Copper deposition in the limbus of the cornea gives rise to the **corneal Kayser-Fleischer ring,** which is a pathognomonic sign.

G. **Tardive dyskinesia** is a syndrome of **repetitive choreic movements affecting the face and trunk,** which result from treatment with phenothiazines, butyrophenones, or metoclopramide.

22

Neurotransmitters

I. IMPORTANT TRANSMITTERS AND THEIR PATHWAYS

A. Acetylcholine (ACh) is the major transmitter of the peripheral nervous system (PNS), neuromuscular junction, parasympathetic nervous system, preganglionic sympathetic fibers, and postganglionic sympathetic fibers that innervate **sweat glands** and **some blood vessels** in skeletal muscles (Figure 22-1). ACh is found in neurons of the basal and visceral motor nuclei in the brain stem and spinal cord. It is also found in the **basal nucleus of Meynert,** which degenerates in **Alzheimer's disease**.

B. Catecholamines. Figure 22-2 shows the biosynthetic pathway for catecholamines. Epinephrine, although a catecholamine, plays an insignificant role as a CNS neurotransmitter. In the body, it is found primarily in the adrenal medulla; in the central nervous system (CNS), it is restricted to small neuronal clusters in the brain stem (medulla).

  1. Dopamine (Figure 22-3) is depleted in patients with Parkinson's disease and is increased in patients with schizophrenia. It has two major receptors: D_1 and D_2.

   a. D_1 **receptors** are postsynaptic and activate adenylate cyclase and are excitatory.

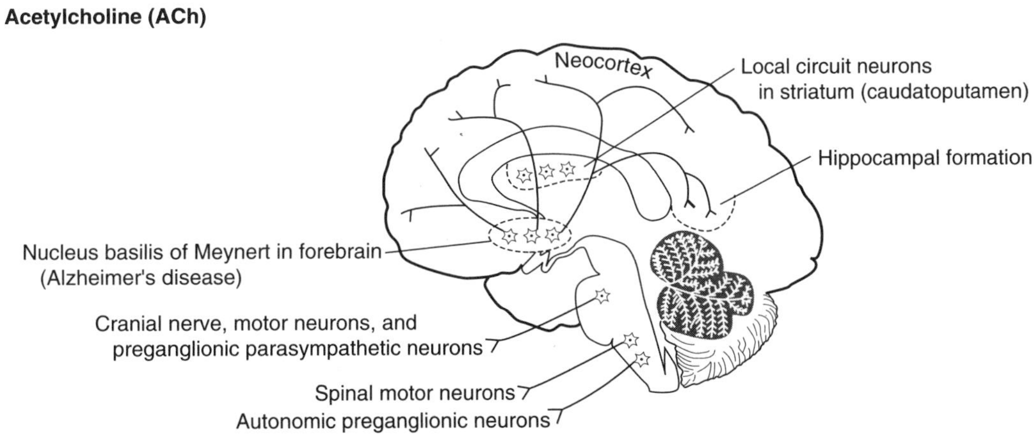

Acetylcholine (ACh)

Figure 22-1. Distribution of acetylcholine (ACh)-containing neurons and their axonal projections. The basal nucleus of Meynert projects to the entire cortex; this nucleus degenerates in patients with Alzheimer's disease. Striatal ACh local-circuit neurons degenerate in patients with Huntington's disease.

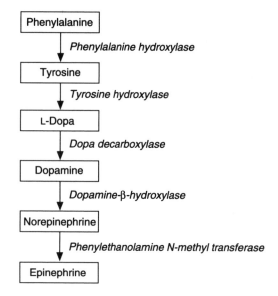

Figure 22-2. Synthesis of catecholamines from phenylalanine. Epinephrine, which is derived from norepinephrine, is found primarily in the adrenal medulla.

b. D_2 **receptors** are both postsynaptic and presynaptic. They inhibit adenylate cyclase and are inhibitory. Antipsychotic drugs block D_2 receptors.

2. **Norepinephrine** (Figure 22-4) is the transmitter of most postganglionic sympathetic neurons. Antidepressant drugs enhance its transmission.

a. Norepinephrine plays a role in **anxiety** states; **panic attacks** are thought to result from paroxysmal discharges from the **locus ceruleus (LC),** where norepinephrinergic neurons are found in the highest concentration. Most postsynaptic receptors of the LC pathway have $ß_1$ and $ß_2$ receptors that activate adenylate cyclase and are excitatory.

Dopamine

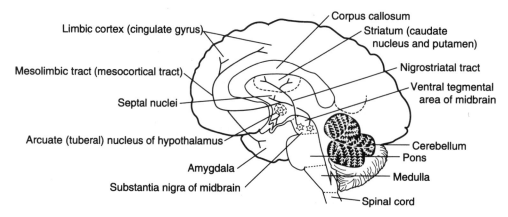

Figure 22-3. Distribution of dopamine-containing neurons and their projections. Two major ascending dopamine pathways arise in the midbrain: the nigrostriatal tract from the substantia nigra and the mesolimbic tract from the ventral tegmental area. In patients with Parkinson's disease, loss of dopaminergic neurons occurs in the substantia nigra and in the ventral tegmental area. Dopaminergic neurons from the arcuate nucleus of the hypothalamus project to the portal vessels of the infundibulum.

Norepinephrine (NE)

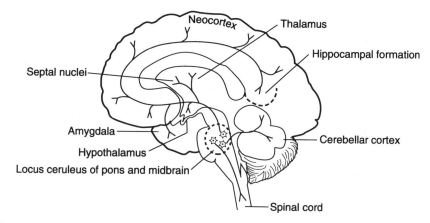

Figure 22-4. Distribution of norepinephrine-containing neurons and their projections. The locus ceruleus, which is located in the pons and midbrain, is the chief source of noradrenergic fibers. The locus ceruleus projects to all parts of the central nervous system (CNS).

  b. The **catecholamine hypothesis of mood disorders** states that reduced norepinephrine activity is related to depression, and that increased norepinephrine activity is related to mania.

C. Serotonin [5-Hydroxytryptamine; (5-HT)] is an indolamine (Figure 22-5). Serotonin neurons are found only in the **raphe nuclei** of the brain stem.

  1. The **permissive serotonin hypothesis** states that reduced 5-HT activity permits reduced levels of catecholamines to cause depression and insomnia, and increased 5-HT activity permits elevated levels of catecholamines to cause mania. Dysfunction of 5-HT may underlie obsessive-compulsive disorder.

  2. Certain **antidepressants** increase 5-HT availability by reducing its reuptake. 5-HT agonists that bind 5-HT_{1A} and those that block 5-HT_{2} have antidepressant properties.

D. Opioid peptides (endogenous opiates) induce responses that resemble those of heroin and morphine.

  1. **Endorphins** include ß-endorphin, which is the major endorphin found in the brain. It is one of the most powerful analgesics known; it is 48 times more potent than morphine. Endorphins are found exclusively in the hypothalamus.

  2. **Enkephalins** are the most widely distributed and abundant opiate peptides. They are found in the highest concentrations in the globus pallidus. Enkephalins coexist with dopamine, γ-aminobutyric acid (GABA), norepinephrine, and acetylcholine. They are co-localized in GABA-ergic pallidal neurons, and they play a role in pain suppression.

  3. **Dynorphins** follow the distribution map for enkephalins.

E. Nonopioid neuropeptides

  1. **Substance P** plays a role in **pain transmission**. It is found in dorsal root ganglion cells, the substantia gelatinosa, and, in its highest concentration, in the substantia nigra. It is co-localized with GABA in the striatonigral tract and plays a role in **movement disorders**. Substance P levels are **reduced in** patients with **Huntington's disease**.

Serotonin (5-HT)

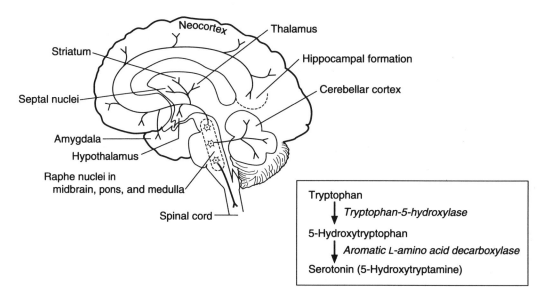

Figure 22-5. Distribution of 5-hydroxytryptamine (5-HT; serotonin)-containing neurons and their projections. Serotonin-containing neurons are found in the nuclei of the raphe. They project widely to the forebrain, the cerebellum, and the spinal cord. The *inset* shows the synthetic pathway of serotonin.

    2. Somatostatin (somatotropin-release inhibiting factor). Somatostatinergic neurons from the anterior hypothalamus project their axons to the median eminence, where somatostatin enters the hypophyseal portal system and **regulates the release of growth hormone (GH) and thyroid-stimulating hormone (TSH)**. The concentration of somatostatin in the neocortex and hippocampus is significantly **reduced in** patients with **Alzheimer's disease**. Striatal somatostatin levels are **increased in** patients with **Huntington's disease**.

F. Amino acid transmitters

    1. Inhibitory amino acid transmitters

        a. GABA (Figure 22-6) is the major inhibitory neurotransmitter of the brain. Purkinje, stellate, basket, and Golgi cells of the cerebellar cortex are GABA-ergic.

            (1) GABA-ergic striatal neurons project to the globus pallidus and the substantia nigra.

            (2) GABA-ergic pallidal neurons project to the thalamus.

            (3) GABA-ergic nigral neurons project to the thalamus.

            (4) GABA receptors (GABA-A and GABA-B) are intimately associated with benzodiazepine-binding sites; benzodiazepines enhance GABA activity.

                (a) GABA-A receptors open chloride channels.

                (b) GABA-B receptors are found on the terminals of neurons using another transmitter (i.e, norepinephrine, dopamine, serotonin). Activation of GABA-B receptors decreases the release of the other transmitter.

        b. Glycine is the major inhibitory neurotransmitter of the spinal cord. It is used by the Renshaw cells of the spinal cord.

γ-Aminobutyric acid (GABA)

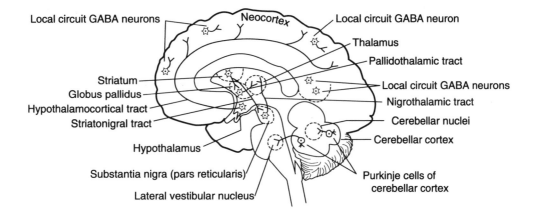

Figure 22-6. Distribution of γ-aminobutyric acid (GABA)-containing neurons and their projections. GABA-ergic neurons are the major inhibitory cells of the central nervous system (CNS). GABA local-circuit neurons are found in the neocortex, hippocampal formation, and cerebellar cortex (Purkinje cells). Striatal GABA-ergic neurons project to the thalamus and the subthalamic nucleus (not shown).

   2. Excitatory amino acid transmitters

      a. Glutamate (Figure 22-7) is the **major excitatory transmitter of the brain**. Neo-cortical glutamatergic neurons project to the striatum, the subthalamic nucleus, and the thalamus.

        (1) Glutamate is the transmitter of the cerebellar granule cells.

        (2) Glutamate is also the transmitter of non-nociceptive, large, primary afferent fibers entering the spinal cord and brain stem.

        (3) Glutamate is the transmitter of the corticobulbar and corticospinal tracts.

Glutamate

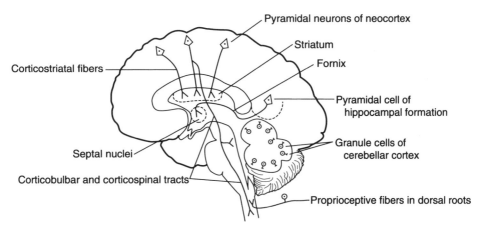

Figure 22-7. Distribution of glutamate-containing neurons and their projections. Glutamate is considered the major excitatory transmitter of the central nervous system (CNS). Cortical glutamatergic neurons project to the striatum; hippocampal and subicular glutamatergic neurons project via the fornix to the septal area and the hypothalamus. The granule cells of the cerebellum are glutamatergic.

b. Aspartate is a major excitatory transmitter of the brain. It is the transmitter of the climbing fibers of the cerebellum (neurons of climbing fibers are found in the inferior olivary nucleus).

c. Behavioral correlates. Glutamate, via its **NMDA** (*N*-methyl-D-aspartate) **receptors,** plays a role in **long-term potentiation** (a memory process) of hippocampal neurons. Glutamate plays a role in **kindling** and subsequent **seizure activity.** Glutamate and its analogs are **neurotoxic** under certain conditions.

II. FUNCTIONAL AND CLINICAL CONSIDERATIONS

A. Parkinson's disease results from degeneration of dopaminergic neurons found in the pars compacta of the substantia nigra. It results in a reduction of dopamine in the striatum and in the substantia nigra (see Chapter 21 III A).

B. Huntington's disease (chorea) results from a loss of ACh- and GABA-containing neurons in the striatum (caudatoputamen). The effect is a loss of GABA in the striatum and substantia nigra (see Chapter 21 III C).

C. Alzheimer's disease results from the degeneration of cortical neurons and cholinergic neurons found in the basal nucleus of Meynert. It is associated with a 60% to 90% loss of choline acetyltransferase in the cerebral cortex. Histologically, Alzheimer's disease is characterized by the presence of neurofibrillary tangles, senile (neuritic) plaques, amyloid substance, granulovacuolar degeneration, and Hirano bodies.

D. Myasthenia gravis is an autoimmune syndrome that occurs in the presence of antibodies to the nicotinic ACh receptor. It is caused by the action of antibodies that reduce the number of receptors in the neuromuscular junction, which results in muscle paresis.

23

Cerebral Cortex

I. INTRODUCTION. The cerebral cortex, the thin, gray covering of both hemispheres of the brain, consists of two types: the neocortex (90%) and the allocortex (10%).

II. THE SIX-LAYERED NEOCORTEX. Layers II and IV of the neocortex are mainly afferent (i.e., receiving); layers V and VI are mainly efferent (i.e., sending).

    A. Layer I is the **molecular** layer.

    B. Layer II is the **external granular** layer.

    C. Layer III is the **external pyramidal** layer. It gives rise to association and commissural fibers and is the major source of corticocortical fibers.

    D. Layer IV is the **internal granular** layer. It receives thalamocortical fibers from the thalamic nuclei of the ventral tier [i.e., ventral posterolateral (VPL) and ventral posteromedial (VPM)]. In the visual cortex (area 17), layer IV receives input from the lateral geniculate body.

    E. Layer V is the **internal pyramidal** layer. It gives rise to corticobulbar, corticospinal, and corticostriatal fibers. It contains the giant pyramidal cells of Betz, which are found only in the motor cortex (area 4).

    F. Layer VI is the **multiform** layer. It is the **major source of corticothalamic fibers**. It gives rise to projection, commissural, and association fibers.

III. FUNCTIONAL AREAS OF THE CEREBRAL CORTEX (Figure 23-1)

    A. Frontal lobe

        1. The **motor cortex (area 4) and premotor cortex (area 6)** are somatotopically organized (Figure 23-2). Destruction of these areas of the frontal lobe results in contralateral spastic paresis.

        2. **Frontal eye field (area 8).** Destruction results in deviation of the eyes to the ipsilateral side.

        3. **Broca's speech area (areas 44 and 45)** is located in the posterior part of the inferior frontal gyrus in the dominant hemisphere (Figure 23-3). Destruction results in an expressive, nonfluent aphasia (Broca's aphasia), in which the patient understands language both written and spoken but cannot articulate speech or write normally.

A

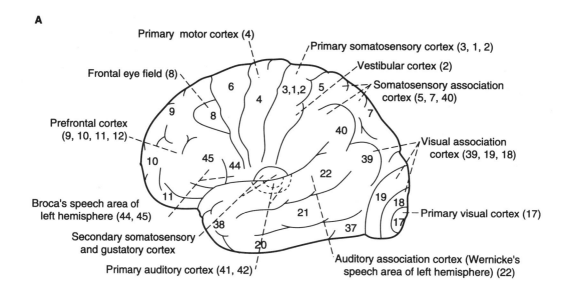

Primary motor cortex (4)

Frontal eye field (8)

Primary somatosensory cortex (3, 1, 2)

Vestibular cortex (2)

Somatosensory association cortex (5, 7, 40)

Prefrontal cortex (9, 10, 11, 12)

Visual association cortex (39, 19, 18)

Broca's speech area of left hemisphere (44, 45)

Primary visual cortex (17)

Secondary somatosensory and gustatory cortex

Primary auditory cortex (41, 42)

Auditory association cortex (Wernicke's speech area of left hemisphere) (22)

B

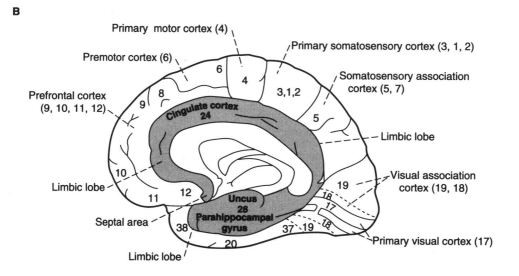

Primary motor cortex (4)

Premotor cortex (6)

Primary somatosensory cortex (3, 1, 2)

Somatosensory association cortex (5, 7)

Prefrontal cortex (9, 10, 11, 12)

Cingulate cortex 24

Limbic lobe

Limbic lobe

Visual association cortex (19, 18)

Septal area

Uncus 28
Parahippocampal gyrus

Primary visual cortex (17)

Limbic lobe

Figure 23-1. Some motor and sensory areas of the cerebral cortex. (*A*) Lateral convex surface of the hemisphere. (*B*) Medial surface of the hemisphere. The numbers refer to the Brodmann brain map, the Brodmann areas.

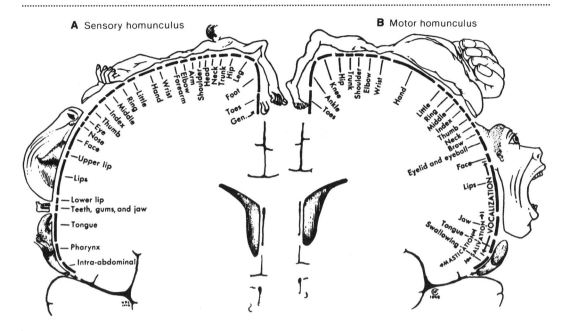

A Sensory homunculus

B Motor homunculus

Figure 23-2. The sensory and motor homunculi. (A) Sensory representation in the postcentral gyrus. (B) Motor representation in the precentral gyrus. (Reprinted with permission from Penfield W and Rasmussen T: *The Cerebral Cortex of Man.* New York, Hafner Publishing, 1968, pp 44 and 57.)

    4. Prefrontal cortex (areas 9–12 and 46–47). Destruction of the anterior two-thirds of the frontal lobe convexity results in deficits in the following functions: concentration, orientation, abstracting ability, judgment, and problem solving. Other frontal lobe deficits are loss of initiative, inappropriate behavior, release of sucking and grasping reflexes, gait apraxia, and sphincteric incontinence. Destruction of the orbital (frontal) lobe results in inappropriate social behavior (e.g., use of obscene language and urinating in public).

B. Parietal lobe

    1. The **sensory cortex (areas 3, 1, and 2)** is somatotopically organized (see Figure 23-1). Destruction of these areas results in contralateral hemihypesthesia and astereognosis.

    2. The **superior parietal lobule (areas 5 and 7).** Destruction of this lobule results in contralateral astereognosis and sensory neglect.

    3. The **inferior parietal lobule of the dominant hemisphere.** Damage to the angular gyrus results in Gerstmann's syndrome, which includes the following deficits:
      a. Right/left confusion
      b. Finger agnosia
      c. Dysgraphia and dyslexia
      d. Dyscalculia
      e. Contralateral hemianopia or lower quadrantanopia

    4. The **inferior parietal lobule of the nondominant hemisphere.** Destruction of this lobule results in:
      a. Topographic memory loss

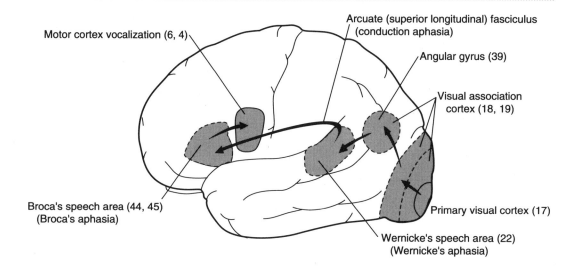

Figure 23-3. Cortical areas of the dominant hemisphere that play an important role in language production. The visual image of a word is projected from the visual cortex (17) to the visual association cortices (18 and 19) and then to the angular gyrus (39). Further processing occurs in Wernicke's speech area (22), where the auditory form of the word is recalled. Via the arcuate fasciculus, this information reaches Broca's speech area (44 and 45), where motor speech programs control the vocalization mechanisms of the precentral gyrus. Lesions of Broca's speech area, Wernicke's speech area, or the arcuate fasciculus result in dysphasias.

    b. Anosognosia

    c. Construction apraxia

    d. Dressing apraxia

    e. Contralateral sensory neglect

    f. Contralateral hemianopia or lower quadrantanopia

C. **Temporal lobe**

  1. The **primary auditory cortex (areas 41 and 42).** Unilateral destruction of these areas of the cortex results in slight loss of hearing. Bilateral loss results in cortical deafness.

  2. **Wernicke's speech area in the dominant hemisphere** is found in the posterior part of the superior temporal gyrus (area 22). Destruction results in a receptive, fluent aphasia (Wernicke's aphasia), in which the patient cannot understand any form of language. Speech is spontaneous, fluent, and rapid but makes little sense.

  3. **Meyer's loop** (see Chapter 17 II F 2) consists of the visual radiations that project to the inferior bank of the calcarine sulcus. Interruption results in a contralateral upper quadrantanopia (pie in the sky).

  4. **Olfactory bulb, tract, and primary cortex** (area 34). Destruction results in ipsilateral anosmia. An irritative lesion (psychomotor epilepsy) of the uncus results in olfactory and gustatory hallucinations.

  5. **Hippocampal cortex (archicortex).** Bilateral lesions result in the inability to consolidate short-term memory into long-term memory; earlier memories are retrievable.

A

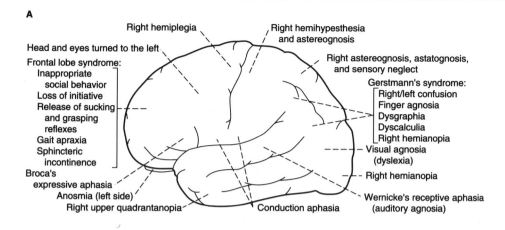

Right hemiplegia

Right hemihypesthesia and astereognosis

Head and eyes turned to the left

Frontal lobe syndrome:
  Inappropriate
    social behavior
  Loss of initiative
  Release of sucking
    and grasping
    reflexes
  Gait apraxia
  Sphincteric
    incontinence

Broca's
  expressive aphasia

Anosmia (left side)

Right upper quadrantanopia

Right astereognosis, astatognosis, and sensory neglect

Gerstmann's syndrome:
  Right/left confusion
  Finger agnosia
  Dysgraphia
  Dyscalculia
  Right hemianopia

Visual agnosia
  (dyslexia)

Right hemianopia

Wernicke's receptive aphasia
  (auditory agnosia)

Conduction aphasia

B

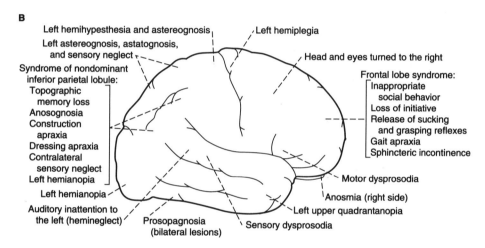

Left hemihypesthesia and astereognosis

Left astereognosis, astatognosis, and sensory neglect

Syndrome of nondominant
  inferior parietal lobule:
  Topographic
    memory loss
  Anosognosia
  Construction
    apraxia
  Dressing apraxia
  Contralateral
    sensory neglect
  Left hemianopia

Left hemianopia

Auditory inattention to
  the left (hemineglect)

Prosopagnosia
  (bilateral lesions)

Left hemiplegia

Head and eyes turned to the right

Frontal lobe syndrome:
  Inappropriate
    social behavior
  Loss of initiative
  Release of sucking
    and grasping reflexes
  Gait apraxia
  Sphincteric incontinence

Motor dysprosodia

Anosmia (right side)

Left upper quadrantanopia

Sensory dysprosodia

C

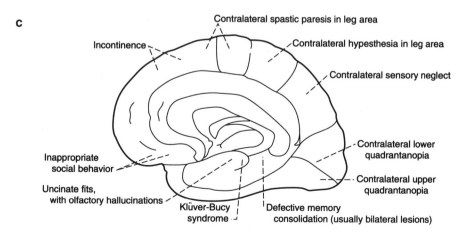

Contralateral spastic paresis in leg area

Incontinence

Contralateral hypesthesia in leg area

Contralateral sensory neglect

Inappropriate
  social behavior

Uncinate fits,
  with olfactory hallucinations

Klüver-Bucy
  syndrome

Contralateral lower
  quadrantanopia

Contralateral upper
  quadrantanopia

Defective memory
  consolidation (usually bilateral lesions)

Figure 23-4. Focal destructive hemispheric lesions and resulting symptoms. (A) Lateral convex surface of the dominant left hemisphere. (B) Lateral convex surface of the nondominant right hemisphere. (C) Medial surface of the nondominant hemisphere.

6. **Anterior temporal lobe.** Bilateral damage in this area results in Klüver-Bucy syndrome, which consists of psychic blindness (visual agnosia), hyperphagia, docility, and hypersexuality.

7. **Inferomedial occipitotemporal cortex.** Bilateral lesions may result in the inability to recognize once-familiar faces (prosopagnosia).

D. Occipital lobe. Bilateral lesions may result in cortical blindness. Unilateral lesions may result in contralateral hemianopia or quadrantanopia.

IV. FOCAL DESTRUCTIVE HEMISPHERIC LESIONS AND SYMPTOMS. Figure 23-4A

shows symptoms of lesions in the dominant hemisphere. Figure 23-4B shows symptoms of lesions in the nondominant hemisphere.

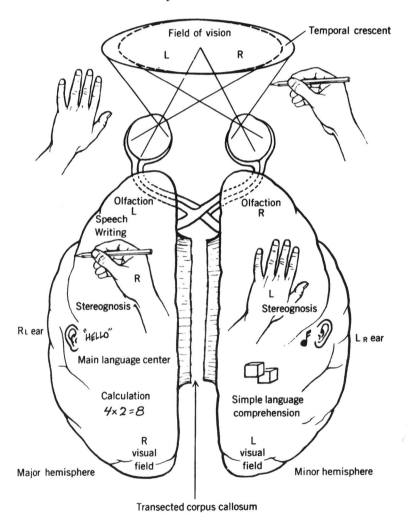

Figure 23-5. Functions of the split-brain after transection of the corpus callosum. Tactile and visual perception is projected to the contralateral hemisphere, olfaction is perceived on the same side, and audition is perceived predominantly in the opposite hemisphere. The left hemisphere is dominant for language; the right hemisphere is dominant for spatial construction and nonverbal ideation. (Reprinted with permission from Noback CR and Demarest RJ: *The Human Nervous System*. Malvern, PA, Lea & Febiger, 1991, p 416.)

V. CEREBRAL DOMINANCE may be determined by the **Wada test,** in which sodium amobarbital (Amytal) is injected into the carotid artery. If the patient becomes aphasic, the anesthetic was given to the dominant hemisphere.

  A. The **dominant hemisphere** is usually the left hemisphere. It is responsible for language, speech, and calculation.

  B. The **nondominant hemisphere** is usually the right hemisphere. It is responsible for three-dimensional or spatial perception and nonverbal ideation. The nondominant hemisphere allows superior recognition of faces.

VI. SPLIT-BRAIN SYNDROME (Figure 23-5) represents a disconnection syndrome that results from **transection of the corpus callosum.**

  A. The **dominant hemisphere** is better at vocal naming.

  B. The **nondominant, mute hemisphere** is better at pointing to a stimulus. Patients are unable to name objects presented to the nondominant visual cortex. Blindfolded patients cannot name objects presented to the nondominant sensory cortex via touch.

  C. **Test** (Figure 23-6). The patient views a composite picture of two half-faces (i.e., a chimeric or hybrid figure), in which the right face is that of a man; the left face is that of a woman. The patient is asked to say what he saw. The patient may respond that he saw a man but, when asked to point to what he saw, he points to the woman.

  D. Patients have **alexia** in the left visual fields (the verbal symbols seen in the right visual cortex have no access to the language centers of the left hemisphere).

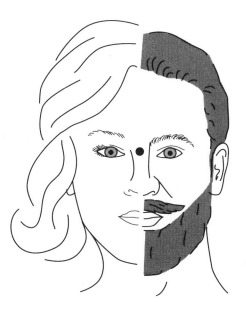

Figure 23-6. Chimeric (hybrid) figure of a face used to examine the hemispheric function of commissurotomized patients. The patient is instructed to fixate on the dot. If the patient is asked verbally to describe what he sees and he says that he sees the face of a man, then the left hemisphere predominates in vocal tasks. If asked to point to the face and he points to the woman, then the right hemisphere predominates in pointing tasks.

Appendix: Table of Cranial Nerves

Cranial nerve	Type	Origin	Function	Course
I—Olfactory	SVA	Bipolar olfactory neurons (in olfactory epithelium in roof of nasal cavity)	Smell (olfaction)	Central axons project to the olfactory bulb via the cribriform plate of the ethmoid bone.
II—Optic	SSA	Retinal ganglion cells	Vision	Central axons converge at the optic disk and form the optic nerve, which enters the skull via the optic canal. Optic nerve axons terminate in the lateral geniculate bodies.
III—Oculomotor				
Parasympathetic	GVE	Edinger-Westphal nucleus (rostral midbrain)	Sphincter muscle of iris; ciliary muscle	Axons exit the midbrain in the interpeduncular fossa, traverse the cavernous sinus, and enter the orbit via superior orbital fissure.
Motor	GSE	Oculomotor nucleus (rostral midbrain)	Superior, inferior, and medial recti muscles; inferior oblique muscle; levator palpebrae muscle	
IV—Trochlear	GSE	Trochlear nucleus (caudal midbrain)	Superior oblique muscle	Axons decussate in superior medullary velum, exit dorsally inferior to the inferior colliculi, encircle the midbrain, traverse the cavernous sinus, and enter the orbit via the superior orbital fissure.
V—Trigeminal				
Motor	SVE	Motor nucleus CN V (mid pons)	Muscles of mastication and tensor tympani muscle	Ophthalmic nerve exits via the superior orbital fissure; maxillary nerve exits via the foramen rotundum; mandibular nerve exits via the foramen ovale; ophthalmic and maxillary nerves traverse the cavernous sinus; GSA fibers enter the spinal trigeminal tract of CN V.
Sensory	GSA	Trigeminal ganglion and mesencephalic nucleus CN V (rostral pons and midbrain)	Tactile, pain, and thermal sensation from the face; the oral and nasal cavities; and the supratentorial dura	
VI—Abducent	GSE	Abducent nucleus (caudal pons)	Lateral rectus muscle	Axons exit the pons from the inferior pontine sulcus, traverse the cavernous sinus, and enter the orbit via the superior orbital fissure.

(appendix cont.)

Cranial nerve	Type	Origin	Function	Course
VII—Facial				
Parasympathetic	GVE	Superior salivatory nucleus (caudal pons)	Lacrimal gland (via sphenopalatine ganglion); submandibular and sublingual glands (via submandibular ganglion)	Axons exit the pons in the cerebellar pontine angle and enter the internal auditory meatus; motor fibers traverse the facial canal of the temporal bone and exit via the stylomastoid foramen; taste fibers traverse the chorda tympani and lingual nerve; GSA fibers enter the spinal trigeminal tract of CN V; SVA fibers enter the solitary tract.
Motor	SVE	Facial nucleus (caudal pons)	Muscles of facial expression; stapedius muscle	
Sensory	GSA	Geniculate ganglion (temporal bone)	Tactile sensation to skin of ear	
Sensory	SVA	Geniculate ganglion	Taste sensation from the anterior two-thirds of tongue (via chorda tympani)	
VIII—Vestibulocochlear	SSA			Vestibular and cochlear nerves join in the internal auditory meatus and enter the brainstem in the cerebellopontine angle; vestibular nerve projects to the vestibular nuclei and the flocculonodular lobe of the cerebellum; cochlear nerve projects to the cochlear nuclei.
Vestibular nerve		Vestibular ganglion (internal auditory meatus)	Equilibrium (innervates hair cells of semicircular ducts, saccule, and utricle)	
Cochlear nerve		Spiral ganglion (modiolus of temporal bone)	Hearing (innervates hair cells of the organ of Corti)	
IX—Glossopharyngeal				Axons exit (motor) and enter (sensory) medulla from the postolivary sulcus; axons exit and enter the skull via jugular foramen; GSA fibers enter the spinal trigeminal tract of CN V; GVA and SVA fibers enter the solitary tract.
Parasympathetic	GVE	Inferior salivatory nucleus (rostral medulla)	Parotid gland (via the otic ganglion)	
Motor	SVE	Nucleus ambiguus (rostral medulla)	Stylopharyngeus muscle	
Sensory	GSA	Superior ganglion (jugular foramen)	Tactile sensation to external ear	
Sensory	GVA	Inferior (petrosal) ganglion (in jugular foramen)	Tactile sensation to posterior third of tongue, pharynx, middle ear, and auditory tube; input from carotid sinus and carotid body	

Cranial nerve	Type	Origin	Function	Course
Sensory	SVA	Inferior (petrosal) ganglion (in jugular foramen)	Taste from posterior third of tongue	
X—Vagal				Axons exit (motor) and enter (sensory) medulla from the postolivary sulcus; axons exit and enter the skull via the jugular foramen; GSA fibers enter the spinal trigeminal tract of CN V; GVA and SVA fibers enter the solitary tract.
Parasympathetic	GVE	Dorsal nucleus of CN X (medulla)	Viscera of the thoracic and abdominal cavities to the left colic flexure [via terminal (mural) ganglia]	
Motor	SVE	Nucleus ambiguus (mid-medulla)	Muscles of the larynx and pharynx	
Sensory	GSA	Superior ganglion (jugular foramen)	Tactile sensation to external ear	
Sensory	GVA	Inferior (nodose) ganglion (in jugular foramen)	Mucous membranes of the pharynx, larynx, esophagus, trachea, and thoracic and abdominal viscera to the left colic flexure	
Sensory	SVA	Inferior (nodose) ganglion (in jugular foramen)	Taste from the epiglottis	
XI—Accessory	SVE			Axons from the cranial division exit the medulla from the postolivary sulcus and join the vagal nerve; axons from spinal division exit the spinal cord, ascend through the foramen magnum, and exit the skull via the jugular foramen.
Motor (cranial)		Nucleus ambiguus (medulla)	Intrinsic muscles of the larynx (except the cricothyroid muscle) via recurrent laryngeal nerve	
Motor (spinal)		Ventral horn neurons C1–C6	Sternocleidomastoid and trapezius muscles	
XII—Hypoglossal	GSE	Hypoglossal nucleus (medulla)	Intrinsic and extrinsic muscles of the tongue (except the palatoglossus muscle)	Axons exit from the preolivary sulcus of the medulla and exit the skull via the hypoglossal canal.